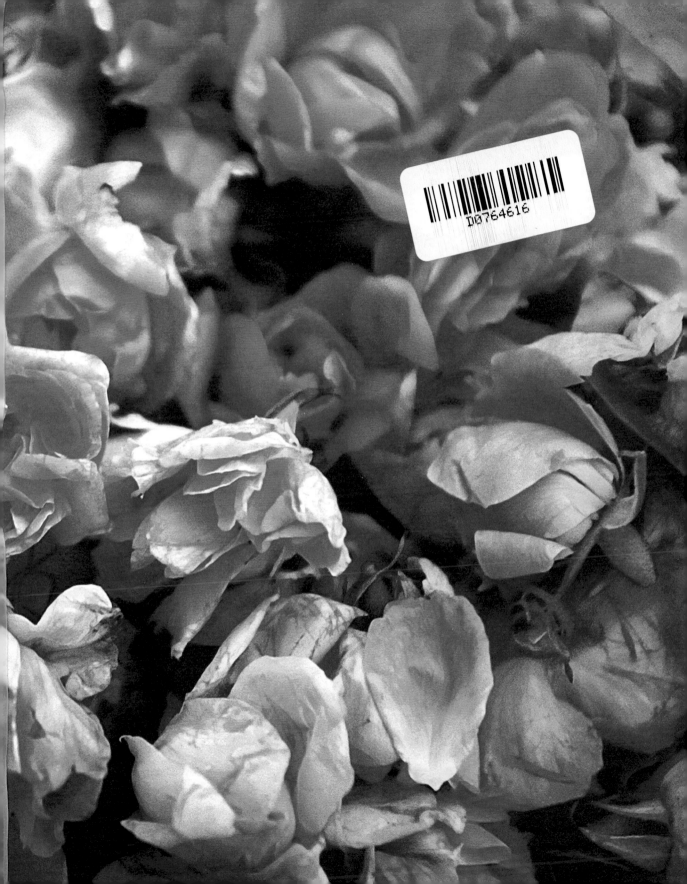

The Organic Pharmacy

The complete guide to natural health and beauty

Margo Marrone

B.Pharm., M.A., L.Hom., M.R.Pharm.S.

DUNCAN BAIRD PUBLISHERS

LONDON

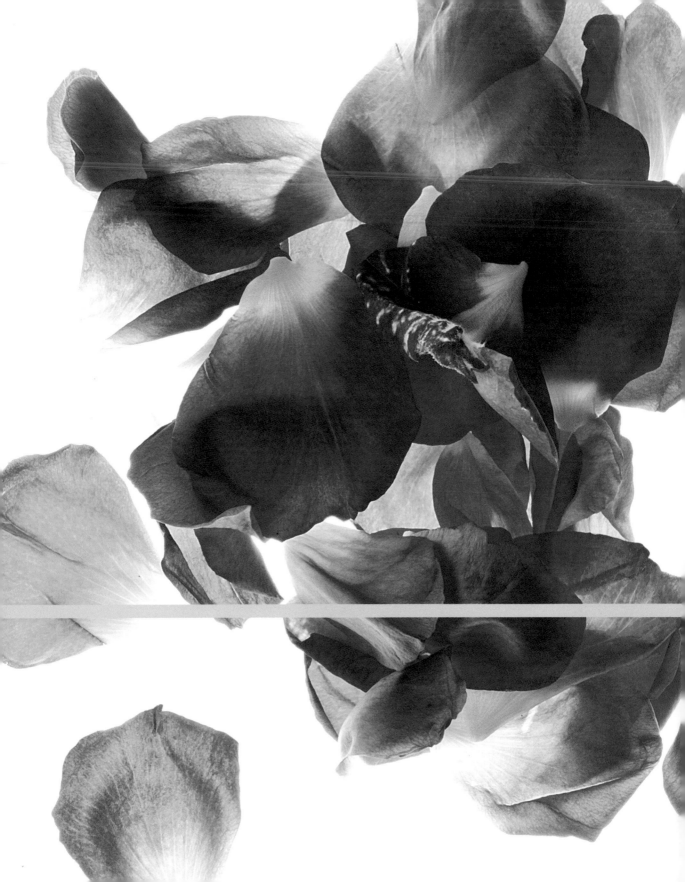

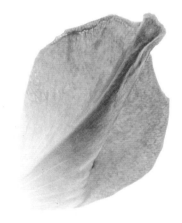

"The Organic
Pharmacy was
the realization
of my dream ...

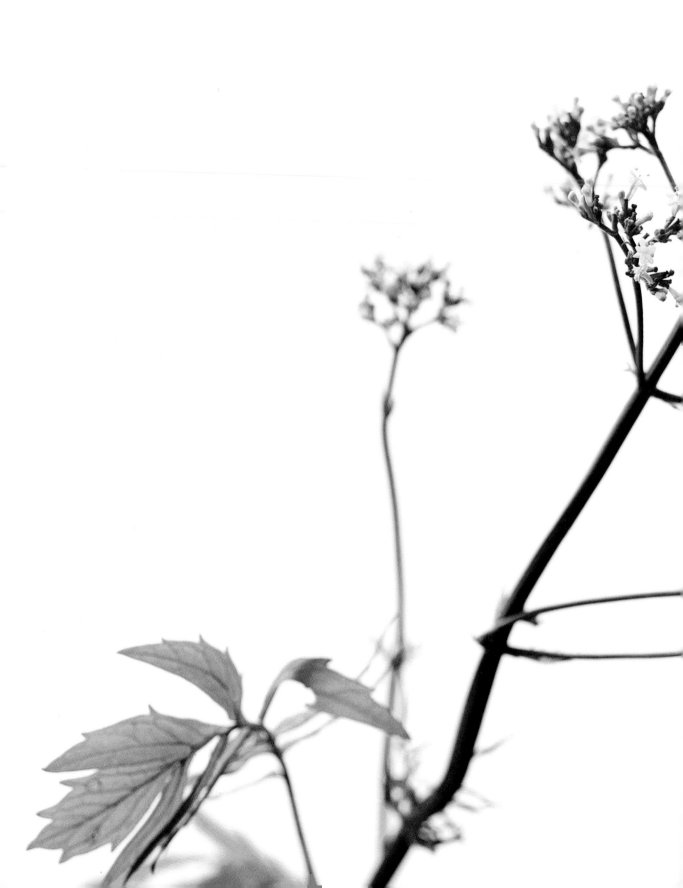

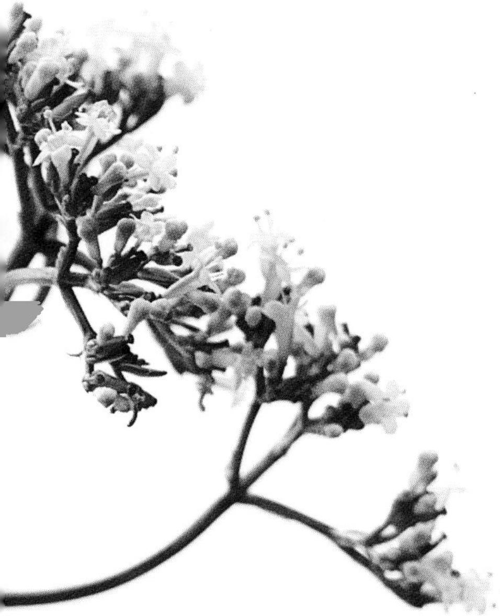

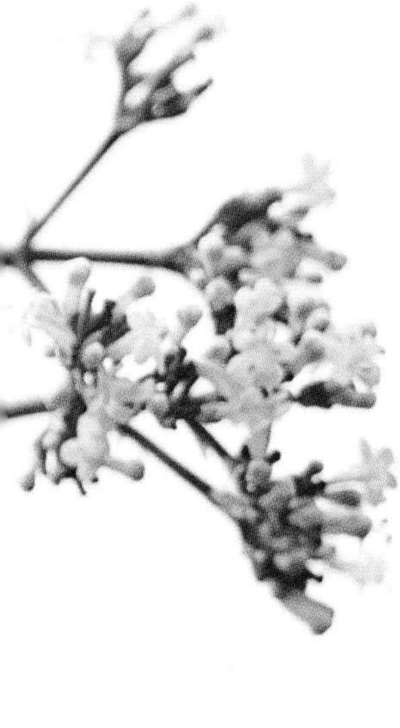

... This book is
my opportunity
to share that
dream with you."

MARGO MARRONE

The Organic Pharmacy
Margo Marrone

Distributed in the USA and Canada by
Sterling Publishing Co., Inc.
387 Park Avenue South
New York, NY 10016-8810

This edition first published in the UK and USA in 2009 by
Duncan Baird Publishers Ltd
Sixth Floor, Castle House
75–76 Wells Street
London W1T 3QH

Managing Editor: Grace Cheetham
Editor: Judy Barratt
Managing Designer: Manisha Patel
Designer: Gail Jones
Commissioned artwork: Wendy Plovmand
Commissioned photography: Toby Scott and Jules Selmes
Picture research: Susannah Stone

Library of Congress Cataloging-in-Publication Data available

ISBN: 978-1-84483-732-8
10 9 8 7 6 5 4 3 2 1

Typeset in Univers
Color reproduction by Colourscan, Singapore
Printed in Malaysia by Imago

For information about custom editions, special sales, premium
and corporate purchases, please contact Sterling Special Sales
Department at 800-805-5489 or specialsales@sterlingpub.com.

Publisher's note:
The information in this book is not intended as a substitute for
professional medical advice and treatment. If you are pregnant or
are suffering from any medical conditions or health problems, it
is recommended that you consult a medical professional before
following any of the advice or practices suggested in this book.
   Duncan Baird Publishers, or any other persons who have been
involved in working on this publication, cannot accept responsibility
for any injuries or damage incurred as a result of following the
information, exercises or therapeutic techniques contained in
this book.

Notes on the recipes:
Unless otherwise stated: use large eggs, fruit and vegetables. Use
fresh ingredients, including herbs. Do not mix metric and imperial
measurements.
1tsp = 5ml, 1tbsp = 15ml, 1 cup = 250ml

contents

introduction

I am often asked why I started The Organic Pharmacy or how I came up with the idea. In truth, there was no "Eureka!" moment, but instead an accumulation of a lifetime of experience, a passion, and an extension of my own lifestyle. I am never a good salesperson unless I truly believe in what I recommend.

For me, it all began when I was 15 with my first job as a Saturday girl in my local pharmacy. I was very fortunate – although I didn't know it at the time – that I was able to experience a traditional pharmacy. Bottle after bottle lined the dispensary shelves, labelled such things as "Belladonna", "Ipecac" and "Peppermint water". As I cleaned each bottle, I wondered what each ingredient did and I watched as clients would come to speak to the pharmacist. He would promptly mix them a custom-made remedy for their cough, sore knee or indigestion. I loved the fact that we knew all our clients' names, treated the whole family, knew their history, and had formed a genuine bond with them. It was at that point I knew pharmacy was for me.

By the time I qualified as a pharmacist five years later, everything had changed and pharmacy had lost that traditional feel, along with the unique customer service I loved so much. My quest for a more natural form of medicine led me to study herbs, aromatherapy and Bach flower remedies, but it wasn't until I began to study homeopathy that I realized I had found what I'd been looking for. As I learned more, I became aware of the concept of organic. And then, with my first pregnancy two years later, I started to take an interest in what was actually contained in the cosmetics that my body was absorbing through my skin and then passing on to my unborn baby. At that point I changed my life and the lives of those around me (the ones who would listen). I haven't looked back since.

The Organic Pharmacy was the realization of my dream: to bring under one roof professional advice, an exceptional, personal service that enables me to form a bond with my clients, and the best products in the world that are free from toxins. This book is my opportunity to share that dream with you.

why organic?

Before I became aware of organic, I shopped at my local supermarket and believed that I led a healthy lifestyle and ate a balanced diet. While I was studying homeopathy, I learned about the quality of food and how the foods we consider to be healthy may not be quite so wholesome after all. For example, previously, I was completely unaware that fruit and vegetables can be sprayed with some of the most toxic and poisonous chemicals in the world; that meat is often pumped with antibiotics and growth hormones; that margarine, touted as the healthier version of butter, is in many cases actually hydrogenated fat – the kind that can give you heart disease; and that salad sold in bags is first soaked in a water–chlorine mix to extend its shelf life. My healthy diet suddenly didn't seem so healthy after all.

As I started to appreciate what healthy eating was really all about, I began to look at food labels. I soon realized that a lot of the products I was buying were full of chemicals: preservatives to prolong the shelf life; artificial colorants to make them look good; artificial flavouring to make them taste better; and cheap, poorly produced ingredients to bring down the costs. It was all there for me to see, but beforehand I had simply trusted in the food I was buying and so I had believed that there was no need to look.

From then on, I started looking at all products, not just food. And to my surprise I found that toxins are everywhere in our lives: from the air we breathe to many of the cosmetics we apply to our faces and bodies. It soon became clear to me that toxicity is a major obstacle to optimum health and we should reduce our exposure to it whenever and wherever we have the opportunity. So, you ask me "Why organic?" I answer that organic ingredients (not just foods) provide the only way to be confident that at least the bulk of the products we buy – from food and drink, to cleaning products and cosmetics – are free from some of the deadliest toxins we know. Organic products mean a healthier lifestyle, which in turn means a healthier body and mind. Plus, organic farming uses less energy and produces less waste than other farming methods, which means that organic is kinder to the environment, too.

the organic pharmacy approach

Natural healing – by eating organic food and using natural, organic medicine – forms a hugely important part of taking control of your life. The benefits include reducing your toxic load, providing more nutrients for your body and helping your environment – all of which serve to improve your overall well-being.

Most people believe that benefiting from natural medicine and alternative remedies is a lengthy process and they will need to wait for many months before they see results. While this may be true for some long-term conditions, in the majority of cases, particularly when it comes to acute illnesses, it is possible to get results quickly and safely. In my work as a homeopathic practitioner, I have seen how, often, the correct homeopathic remedy can work to relieve symptoms within minutes – and, by adding herbs and supplements to the prescription, the root cause can be treated even faster.

It is the philosophy of finding the right remedy at the right time for the right person – as well as an approach that combines homeopathy, herbs and supplements with good nutrition – that underpins The Organic Pharmacy model for health and vitality. However, The Organic Pharmacy approach isn't just as simple as giving a remedy. Before I make up any prescription, I ask people to assess their potential toxicity. Almost everyone we see at The Organic Pharmacy has toxins accumulated in their body, which prevents the homeopathic remedies from working as quickly as they might. Detoxification is the cornerstone of all my treatments, because it encourages the body to shed its toxic load – with amazing results. Often, some fifty percent of my clients' symptoms will disappear just by doing the detox, and we take care of the rest using the combined approach to treatment.

Several recent reports have criticized detoxification, but there are studies proving that, if performed properly, it can have remarkable and long-lasting benefits. The Organic Pharmacy detox program (see pp.46–55) has been specifically developed to suit modern lifestyles and I encourage everyone to follow it at least four times a year.

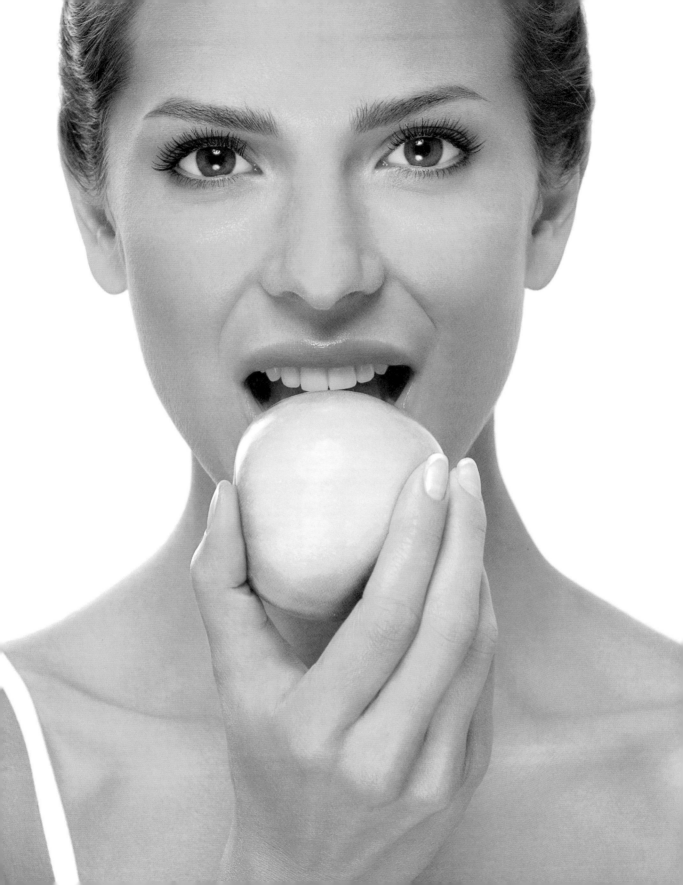

how the treatments work

Your body is made up of several highly complex, interconnected systems that work around the clock to keep you healthy. Fundamental to good health is ensuring these systems are not overloaded with toxins. The treatments I've selected for you in this book aim to maintain the synergy, harmony and balance of your body's systems in order to optimize health. Over the following pages, I'll take you through each of my treatment techniques, to give you a sense of how each works on your body. But, before I do, it's important to give you an overview of the body's systems so that you can apply this knowledge to how you approach my treatments.

THE MAIN BODY SYSTEMS

THE IMMUNE SYSTEM Comprising a series of both internal and external protective measures, your immune system is your body's warrior against invading pathogens, such as bacteria and viruses. The skin – including your internal (epithelial) skin that lines your lungs and gut – gives a first line of defence that is supported by secretions such as hydrochloric acid in the stomach and by the immune cells (such as lymphocytes). The other parts of your body involved in immunity are the thymus, spleen, and lymphatic system. Herbs are wonderful friends to the immune system: in particular, they act as antibacterials and antivirals, and they boost the body's production of immune cells. Nutrients also play a vital role: for example, vitamins C and A have a direct antiviral action, and they also help with detoxification and the production of specific antibodies.

THE DIGESTIVE SYSTEM A healthy digestive system ensures that your cells maximize their uptake of essential nutrients, eliminates toxins effectively from your body and establishes the right balance of good and bad bacteria in your gut (see pp.94–95). In addition, the digestive system is responsible for regulating the body's acid–alkali balance. The body functions best in an alkaline environment. The more acidic your body becomes, the more unwell you feel and the more prone you are to illness. There are many factors that make your body acidic, including your natural metabolism, which

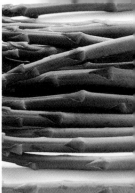

produces acidic by-products that your body then needs to neutralize. Food provides you with the tools to control this balance, and for optimum health my basic rule of thumb is to eat a diet that is made up of eighty percent alkali-forming foods and twenty percent acid-forming foods. I've devised the following lists to help you.

ALKALI-FORMING FOODS
• asparagus • avocados • beetroot (beet) • broccoli • Brussels sprouts • celery • corn • courgettes (zucchini) • garlic • grapefruit • green beans • honey • lemons • lettuce • limes • mangoes • mushrooms • okra • onions • parsley • papayas • raisins • raw spinach • soy products • squash • sweet potato • watermelon

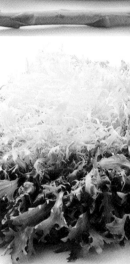

ACID-FORMING FOODS
• alcohol • beans • buckwheat • chickpeas (garbanzos) • cocoa • coffee • cranberries • eggs • flour-based products • lentils • meat • mustard • noodles • pasta • pepper • poultry • shellfish • sugar • tea • vinegar

The following are low-level acid-forming foods that are fine eaten in moderation:
• butter • cheeses • dried fruits • grains • nuts and seeds

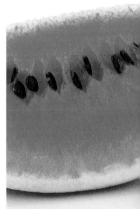

THE CIRCULATORY SYSTEM A healthy circulation is vital to bring oxygen and nutrients to cells and to take away waste products so that cells can function optimally. Through the various treatments, I aim to boost the levels of oxygen in your blood and to make your blood's transportation of nutrients as efficient as possible. This is what I mean when I say that a treatment needs to increase or boost your circulation. The result will be not only healthier insides, but beautiful skin, too.

DETOXIFICATION Almost all diseases and many skin conditions are at least to some degree caused or worsened by toxicity and so detoxification is the cornerstone of almost all of my treatments. A clean body allows nutrients and oxygen to get to cells through improved circulation and allows herbs and homeopathic remedies to act much more swiftly and efficiently to promote both health and beauty.

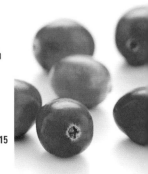

the homeopathy core

Just as every human body is made up of a unique energy, every animal, plant and mineral also has a unique, energetic signature. Taking this one step further, every disease has a unique signature, too, and this signature imprints itself on you when you are ill. Most of the time, your body can cure itself, but at other times it gets stuck and needs outside impetus to encourage proper healing. At its simplest, homeopathy aims to stimulate the body's energy in conjunction with that of the homeopathic remedy to stamp out the energy of the disease and so restore health.

HOW HOMEOPATHY WORKS

The principle that underlies all homeopathic treatment is that a natural substance that produces in your body symptoms similar to those of the particular disease helps your body to cure the disease. When the remedy magnifies the symptoms of the disease, your body's immune system is tricked into thinking that the disease has worsened, so it works harder to fight it off – and therefore you overcome the disease more quickly.

THE ENERGY OF REMEDIES

Homeopathy uses plants, minerals, animals – in fact, almost any substance – as its starting material. This material is diluted in a systematic way to "release" and make available the energy of that material in a water medium. The energy is then made more powerful through a process of dilution and succussion (violent shaking). It is the job of a homeopath to match the energy of the remedy to the energy of the disease. The closer the match, the faster the cure. This is why a homeopath might prescribe a combination of remedies for only one illness. Each remedy in the combination will tackle a particular aspect or symptom of the disease so that (ideally) the whole combination treats the whole disease. The energy of the remedy works best when the body is toxin-free, as the immune system and systems of elimination need to work at their optimum levels to fight illness. And because it works at such an energetic level, homeopathy brings about not only physical cures in your body's systems and your skin, but emotional cures, too.

CHOOSING AND BUYING HOMEOPATHIC REMEDIES

You can buy homeopathic remedies in all good health-food stores and homeopathic pharmacies. They are supplied as lactose tablets, pillules, powder or granules and in different potencies. The more dilute a remedy, the stronger it is and the higher its potency. For example, a 6c potency has been diluted 600 times; a 30c potency, 3,000 times and so on. Weaker remedies are diluted tens of times (they are less dilute), so the potency is given as, for example, 6x.

For each homeopathic remedy I've selected in this book, I've given a suitable potency. However, bear in mind that as homeopathy works with your body's own energy, remedy combinations should really be tailored to your symptoms. In the book, I've given remedies that I've seen work at a general level, but for the best effects nothing can beat a personal consultation with a registered homeopath (your country's official society of homeopaths will have a list of accredited practitioners near you).

HOW TO TAKE HOMEOPATHIC REMEDIES

The standard dosage for a homeopathic remedy is two pillules, which you should suck or chew like sweets (don't swallow them or take them with water). Take the remedies away from meals – this means at least ten minutes before or after you eat. Finally, take all the remedies that I recommend, not only those that seem relevant – the combination will cover several of the typical symptoms specific to the disease.

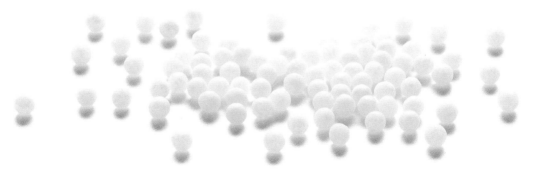

where do herbs fit in?

For me, herbs provide invaluable support for homeopathic treatment and I always prescribe a mix of herbal remedies (usually up to five of them) to assist the recovery process. When I make up a prescription for a client, I often use herbs to improve the body's ability to detoxify, as well as to try to optimize the functioning of its various systems so that they are efficient and effective, creating good health and great skin. In essence, herbs support all the body's organs to allow the immune, reproductive, lymphatic, respiratory, circulatory and nervous systems to work at their best.

THE IMPORTANCE OF HERBAL REMEDIES

Our first medicines were herbs. Long before we ever thought to take a pill, our ancestors – all over the world – were finding remedies in the landscape around them. Since these ancient beginnings, scientific research has proven beyond doubt that the active constituents in plants can have medicinal qualities. With this knowledge, thinking we know better than nature, we have set about extracting these constituents, often replicating them synthetically to make modern medicines. However, in doing so, I believe we missed the point. Herbal remedies are effective because all the active constituents in a herb work in synergy to provide a "whole" cure – often without the

using herbal tinctures

A herbal tincture is made by steeping dried or fresh herbs in alcohol. To be safe, I recommend you buy ready-made commercial tinctures, rather than trying to make your own, as commercial versions will have been manufactured using specific water-to-alcohol ratios for each herb to guarantee specific therapeutic activity. Organic herbal tinctures use organic alcohol and organically grown herbs – for all the same reasons it's better to eat organic foods, it's better to use organic tinctures whenever you can.

side effects of conventional medicines. Taking out just one or two active constituents for a specific purpose undermines the original herb's overall healing capability.

CHOOSING AND BUYING HERBAL REMEDIES

It sounds trite, but with herbs (as with most things), you get what you pay for. Buy the most expensive remedies you can afford, always from organic sources (see p.20). Tincture form is best (see box, opposite), which most good health-food stores and pharmacies will stock. If you are unable to get hold of a tincture, you can use a herbal tea instead. This is called an infusion and it is not as strong as a tincture and so will not have the same healing power, but it will offer some relief.

HOW TO TAKE HERBAL REMEDIES

The standard dosage for most of the conditions in this book is 15 drops of tincture taken in a little water or juice, three times a day. A little water or juice means about 20ml (4 tsp) – just a little in the bottom of a glass. For acute ailments, such as a sore throat or ear infection, it may be necessary to take your tincture remedy more than three times a day – up to five or six times. Follow the dosage advice I've given for each condition. The standard dosage for a herbal infusion is one cup, three times a day, unless your condition requires more frequent relief, as with tinctures.

For acute conditions, stop taking your remedy a few days after you feel better. And whether your condition is chronic or acute, unless it is under the close supervision of a practitioner and medical doctor, never take herbs for more than two to three weeks at a time. If your condition is chronic, have a week's break and then resume for another two to three weeks before breaking again; resuming again if you need to. The break gives your body time to find its equilibrium – in case you don't need the herbs any more – and prevents your system from becoming desensitized to the active ingredients. Some herbs are not suitable for long-term use, so always check with a practitioner.

If you have any reactions to the herbs you take, talk to your practitioner. Some reactions are good signs – indicating that your condition is abating and that the herbs are doing their job. However, on rare occasions you may have an adverse reaction and your practitioner will be able to advise you accordingly.

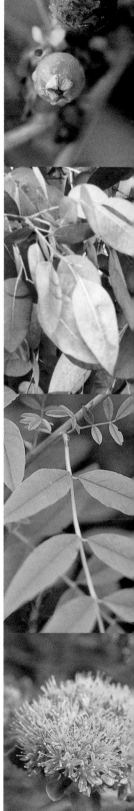

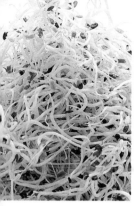

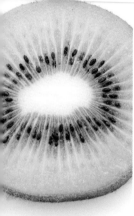

nutrition and supplements

Vitamins, minerals, trace elements and essential fats – your body needs a range of nutrients to function properly. Without them, all the body's systems suffer, especially your immunity, making you more susceptible to illness, and your skin. In an ideal world, you would eat all the right foods in all the right quantities to give you the optimum nutrition your body needs. However, less time to spend cooking coupled with poor-quality soil (and so fewer nutrients in food), mean that your nutritional intake from foods is not nearly good enough – and this is why taking supplements is a necessity for optimum health.

CHOOSING AND BUYING FOOD

The quality of the food that you eat has an enormous impact on your health (see pp.33–35). One of the most important aspects of what I do is talking to my clients about what good nutrition means and how important it is to buy fresh, quality produce that has been organically produced, and to steer clear of processed and packaged foods.

Each of my treatment programs has a section on nutritional advice. Sometimes this advice encourages you to eat certain foods; sometimes it encourages you to steer clear of certain foods. It is always relevant that, as well as being organic, the food you eat should be fresh and seasonal. So much nutrition is lost in travelling times for foods – as soon as a fruit or vegetable is picked from a plant or out of the soil, it begins to lose its nutritional value. If you eat seasonally, preferably from local suppliers, you can help to ensure that what you eat is as fresh as possible, and therefore at its most nutritious.

CHOOSING AND BUYING SUPPLEMENTS

Whenever I treat a client, I prescribe him or her with the necessary supplements to help bring the body back into balance and promote self-healing. However, in order for supplements to help the healing process, it is essential they are of the best quality possible. Just as with herbs, you get what you pay for and I strongly recommend you buy the best-quality supplements you can afford.

YOUR DAILY SUPPLEMENT REGIME

Even during times of good health, I recommend a daily supplement regime to ensure your body is always fighting fit. The following supplements are those I think it is essential to take every day. You will see some of them come up time and again in the treatment programs to help boost the body's systems during periods of illness, but below I recommend taking them daily at a standard dosage, which you can then boost when you need to. (If you find it hard to swallow capsules, empty the contents into a small glass of juice, and drink.)

ANTIOXIDANTS A combined antioxidant supplement helps to neutralize free-radical damage in your body. Free radicals are the maverick atoms that destroy healthy cells, thereby contributing to disease and speeding up the aging process.
DOSAGE Two capsules, daily.

ESSENTIAL FATTY ACIDS AND B-COMPLEX VITAMINS This combined supplement helps your body to generate new cells, lower cholesterol and high blood pressure, regulate brain function and reduce inflammation in the body.
DOSAGE Two capsules, daily.

PHYTONUTRIENTS Take a combined phytonutrients supplement to boost your green foods (see p.192). The chlorophyll in green foods is a wonderful detoxifier.
DOSAGE Two capsules, daily.

PROBIOTICS These are the friendly or "good" bacteria that keep your digestion healthy.
DOSAGE Two billion, daily.

MAKING THE MOST OF YOUR HEALTHY BODY

Although nutrition plays a vital role in your health, for me health is not just about eating well and staying clear of disease. I believe every person has a purpose in life – something that makes them passionate and full of a child-like enthusiasm for everything they do. Optimum nutrition will help to keep your body healthy; optimum attitude will help to boost the health of your mind and emotions. If you have a passion for something or are simply bursting with energy to do something, make the most of it. Indulge in your passions and face each day filled with optimism.

how to use this book

Young or old, man or woman, my unique approach to optimum health and beauty is available to everyone. At The Organic Pharmacy we treat between two and three thousand clients a year, all of whom are looking for an effective, quick and simple approach to optimum health. I hope the advice and treatments outlined in this book will help you to overcome a host of common ailments and generally set you on the path to feeling better on the inside and looking better on the outside, too.

THE DETOX

Whatever your condition or ailment, I strongly recommend you start your treatment program with my easy-to-follow ten-day detox program. I've made it as accessible as possible, so that it's easy to fit in with even the busiest lifestyle.

THE TREATMENT PROGRAMS

Look up your condition in the relevant chapters and follow the treatment program carefully to help you kickstart and support your body's own healing powers. You will find that individual remedies may be recommended for more than one ailment, owing to their large sphere of action. However, before you take any herbs or supplements, check the tables on pages 202–207 for a list of contraindications – that is, reasons why that remedy might not be suitable (for example, if you are pregnant or on certain medication). If you are in any doubt at all as to the suitability of any remedy, either for you or your child, consult a qualified practitioner before you use it. Remember always to follow the three-tier approach of herbs, homeopathy and supplements.

      Every treatment program also offers nutritional advice, giving you information on some of the most nutrient-rich foods to help to fight that particular condition. Try to use them in cooking as much as you can to speed your recovery. Fresh, organic produce is essential at all times, and also try to avoid junk and processed foods (see pp.34–35). I've given specific foods to avoid where I feel they can have a particularly detrimental effect on your health with regard to the specific condition.

about the star ingredients

Nature and its plants are incredible. In order to protect themselves from infection, they produce compounds that are antifungal, antibacterial, antiviral, antioxidant and healing (to repair damage to their own cells). They also produce myriad nutrients. What fascinates me about the plants I use to make my remedies, is the incredible diversity of their action, their potency and their affinity with the body.

Throughout this book, in relevant places, you will find special pages for six "star ingredients". These are the ingredients in cosmetics and remedies that have particularly notable health-giving properties – the ingredients you should look for whenever you need to take particular care of yourself. They are:
• Propolis (pp.72–73) • Aloe vera (pp.106–107) • Calendula (pp.126–127)
• St John's Wort (pp.138–139) • Rose-hip seed oil (pp.150–151) • Rose (pp.200–201)

TREATING CHILDREN

As well as the chapter on childhood illnesses, throughout the book conditions affecting children have feature boxes that adapt adult treatments for growing bodies. Two pills, sucked like sweets, is the standard child dosage of homeopathic remedies. For herbs, the dosage is five drops of tincture in a tablespoon of water or juice.

STAYING SAFE

The treatment programs in this book cannot replace the advice of your own therapist or doctor. Nevertheless, followed carefully (see also tables, pp.202–207), they are perfectly safe. Read pages 16–21 on how to administer homeopathy, herbs and supplements, and for general dosages. Individual dosages are given in the programs themselves.

A NOTE ON THE PICTURES

Relevant plants and foods are illustrated throughout the book. There are visual indexes on pages 208–210 to help you identify them.

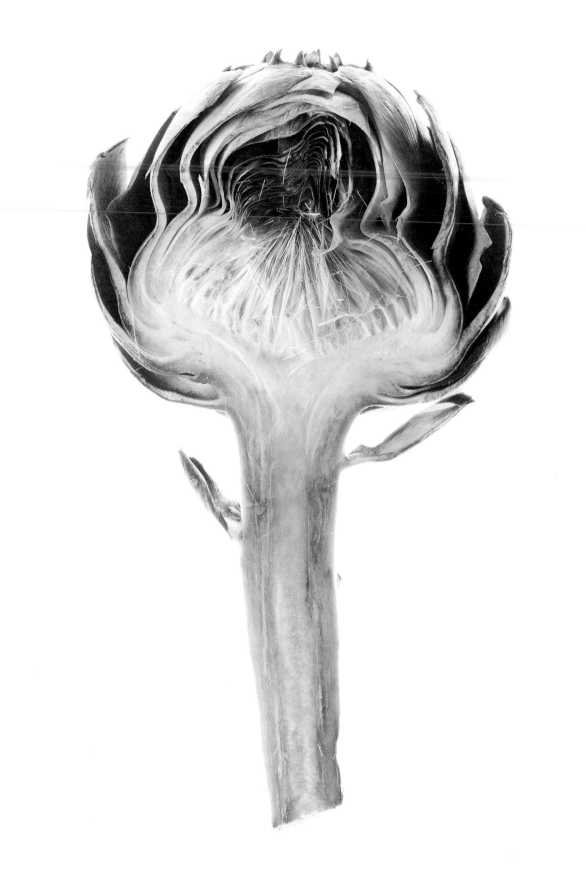

CHAPTER 1

cleansing your body

For some of us, the mere mention of the word detox conjures up images of fasting, starvation, suffering and having to "give up" our favourite foods, and even our most treasured habits. Paradoxically, though, in the vast majority of us, the word detox conjures up images of health, vitality and looking good – which are exactly the reasons why so many of us attempt to carry it out.

A considerable number of the health plans you come across in magazines and books include a two-day or weekend detox. However, my view on these short detoxes is that they just don't give your body enough time for the good work to start properly, meaning that your system gets confused. In order to achieve longlasting, even remarkable results from a detox, the program you follow has to last at least between seven and ten days. Only after this longer period will your great work take root.

I developed the program in this chapter in The Organic Pharmacy clinic and it is specifically tailored to fit in with everyday life. I want you to be able to detox within the parameters of your normal existence, without having to make drastic changes to your lifestyle. However, I also want you to adopt some really fantastic, long-term changes for the better. Use the program to look at every aspect of your life. Let it encourage you to slow down, rest, get rid of bad habits, and enjoy.

left: artichoke (*Cynara scolymus*)

the why, who, what and how of detox

Over the past sixty years, we have seen a tremendous increase in the use of chemicals in all types of industry, including farming. This has brought with it a proliferation of toxins. Pesticides and herbicides that were virtually unknown seventy years ago are now widely used on our crops. Despite the fact that most of us are fastidious about cleaning our homes, cars, clothes and so on, few of us pay attention to cleansing ourselves – at least on the inside – even though inner cleansing has untold benefits for beauty as well as health. Over the years, the debris of everyday toxins accumulates in your blood, liver, lungs, gut and, in fact, all your body's cells. The process of detoxification enables your body to rid itself of these and other unwanted chemicals, including those your body produces by itself (see p.38).

WHO NEEDS TO DETOX?

Anyone who experiences some of the following symptoms may be adversely affected by toxicity and will benefit from undergoing a detox progam. For obvious reasons, the more symptoms you experience, the more urgently your system needs your help.

• age (liver) spots • bad breath • coated tongue • digestive problems (including indigestion, bloating, IBS, candida, constipation) • dull hair and skin • excess weight • headaches • irritability or mood swings • premature aging • tired eyes • tiredness • skin disorders (including acne, eczema, psoriasis, allergies) • sluggish metabolism

When your body is overloaded with toxins, much of your energy is spent on trying to eliminate the toxins rather than on enabling you to live life to the fullest. Additional pressures such as stress, insomnia and emotional problems can aggravate the symptoms of toxic overload, because the body's energies are redirected to deal with your levels of stress, instead of concentrating on the process of detoxification. This is why problems such as eczema and acne often get worse when you are under stress.

THE RESULTS OF A DETOX

Once you have completed your detox, your body will feel and look great – and people will notice. You should experience:

• clear, glowing skin • fresh breath and a clear tongue • good gut health • shiny hair • weight loss • a more alert mind • happier moods • fewer signs of aging • bright eyes • higher energy • better sleep • generally improved health

In addition, your digestive system will be better able to absorb nutrients from foods and supplements – creating a cycle of health. With better nutrition, your body will manage your exposure to environmental chemicals such as those in cigarette smoke and industrial pollution, and you'll be less likely to suffer from reactive or allergic responses.

HOW TO ACHIEVE THE OPTIMUM DETOX

First of all it's really important to keep your detox safe. If you are generally in good health and not taking any regular medication, there is no reason why my detox plan won't work wonders on your body, mind and beauty. However, I would always advise that you consult your doctor or other healthcare practitioner before you embark upon any detox program, just to make sure your body is up to the challenge of cleansing.

There are a couple of circumstances under which you need to take special care. If you are pregnant now isn't the time to cleanse (although a detox can be great for your pre-pregnancy health). If you are on multiple prescription medications, do the detox only under the close supervision of a physician, homeopath or nutritionist, who can monitor your progress carefully. Although detox can, in the long run, be highly energizing, initially it can make you feel tired and depleted. For these reasons, avoid detox if you suffer from a terminal or chronic illness.

Once you are sure that you are up for the challenge of detox, generally speaking, the process involves two main steps. First, you need to identify and reduce your individual toxic load; and second, you need to give your body the tools to eliminate stored toxins. Your body has all sorts of amazing systems that evolution has put in place to ensure that it detoxifies effectively. We explore these next.

how your body detoxifies

In order to really appreciate the need for detox – to be able to visualize what's happening in your body and to get motivated – I want you to know about the main organs and systems that your body uses to detoxify. The liver, kidneys, intestines, skin, lymphatic system, and lungs all play vital roles in keeping your body toxin-free.

THE LIVER (**a**)

Your liver filters your blood to remove bacteria, as well as fat-soluble toxins, many of which you get from your food. This fantastic organ metabolizes these toxins to make them water-soluble, so they can be flushed out of your system via your kidneys in your urine, or in your bile (which forms part of your stool). Your liver also produces enzymes that break down toxins that come from the air, from your food and water, and through your skin, and prepares them for your body to expel in the urine and bile, too. In an overloaded liver, all these processes slow down and health-sapping toxins accumulate in your blood, causing not only illness but also skin problems (see below). One of the main aims of my ten-day detox program is to reduce your liver's load.

THE KIDNEYS (**b**)

Your kidneys receive the water-soluble toxins from your liver and flush them out in your urine. They also filter toxins directly from your blood, keep your blood alkaline (see pp.14–15) and eliminate excess salt from your body (which in turn keeps your blood-fluid levels constant and so doesn't force your heart to overwork). My detox helps with all these processes and so relieves the pressure on your kidneys.

THE SKIN (**c**)

When the liver and kidneys are overloaded, the skin – the largest of all your organs – provides detoxification back-up by expelling toxins through sweat. However, by-products of this are often blemishes or tired-looking skin. Think of my detox program as an essential part of your long-term beauty plan to achieve a blemish-free glow.

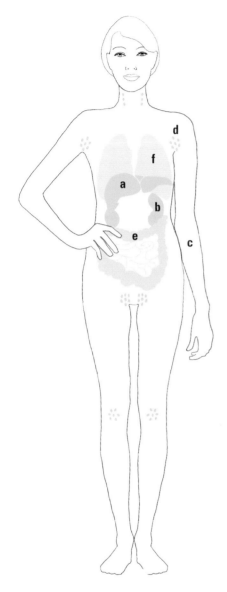

LYMPHATIC DRAINAGE (**d**)

Part of the immune system, a clear fluid called lymph removes toxins, bacteria and other organisms from the body's cells and deposits them in the blood for elimination, at sites called lymph nodes. With no pump of its own, lymphatic drainage relies upon breathing and muscle contraction to move lymph around the body. Use the breathing and stretching exercises in the Detox Toolkit (see p.41) to help its work.

THE INTESTINES (**e**)

Your intestines are the place where you absorb nutrients from your food, but they are also where your body is cleansed of toxins. If you have a poor diet, or you use drugs or drink too much alcohol, you can damage your digestive tract so that decaying food remains in your gut to cause autointoxication – or self-poisoning. Your bloodstream may then reabsorb the toxins, causing all the symptoms of toxicity (see p.26).

The other important thing about your intestines is their balance of good and bad bacteria. The good keeps the bad in check and synthesizes vitamins A, B and K (making them useable for the body), helps the body to digest lactose (milk sugar), and produces natural antibiotics to help to fight infection and break down toxic waste. My detox will optimize the delicate balance of good and bad bacteria in your gut, to make sure that you are in the best digestive health.

THE LUNGS (**f**)

You may breathe in toxins through your lungs, but these amazing machines also expel toxins. Breathe deeply and exhale fully (see p.41 for advice on how) to maximize the cleansing effect.

reducing your toxic load

Simply in the course of living a normal life, the body is bombarded with toxins and so the first step in any detox program must be to reduce the number of toxins you encounter day to day. There are four main ways by which your body is exposed to and absorbs toxins: through the air you breathe, through the water you drink, through the food you eat, and through the products you use on and in your body (in the form of cosmetics and medicines) and in your home (as cleaning products).

Over the following pages, we will look at each of these main sources of toxicity and I will give you practical advice on how you can reduce your exposure to them using safe, natural, effective alternatives. These alternatives are your first steps to becoming as toxin-free as you possibly can be.

THE AIR YOU BREATHE

It's not just motor exhaust fumes, industrial emissions, and dust from construction sites that pollute the air that you (and I and our children) breathe – artificial fragrances such as air fresheners, candles, perfumes, cosmetics and room sprays also send chemicals into the atmosphere for all of us to breathe in. Cleaning products and garden insecticides alone can expose us to between three and four hundred volatile chemicals (that is, chemicals that can cause a reaction in the body) every day.

Most product manufacturers have undertaken minimum amounts of testing on the respiratory effects of fragrance materials even though many of them are organic compounds that can easily affect, among other things, the respiratory system. In addition, many artificial fragrances are neurotoxic (they attack our nervous system), which can cause irritability, allergies and – once again – breathing difficulties. Chemicals present in air fresheners and other perfumed products can irritate the eyes and the mucous membranes of our respiratory tract. They often cause skin reactions. The chemical g-Terpinene, which is present in some air fresheners, can induce asthma and central-nervous-system disorders, such as epilepsy.

avoiding heavy metals

Heavy metals – metals that have a high density and may be toxic – mostly enter your body via food, drinking water, and air, as well as through cigarette smoke. Some of these metals, including cobalt, copper and zinc, are known as "trace elements" and these are essential to your body to maintain its metabolism. Others, including aluminium, lead and mercury, can lead to poisoning when they bioaccumulate – that is, when they are taken up and stored faster in the body than the body can break them down or excrete them. To reduce your exposure to unwanted heavy metals:

• Avoid aluminium-based deodorants and sun creams.

• Use stainless steel cooking utensils.

• Ask your dentist for white fillings, instead of mercury-based ones.

• Use only filtered water for all cooking and drinking. Heavy metals can enter water supplies through industrial and consumer waste, and even from "acid rain", which breaks down in the soil and releases heavy metals into streams, lakes, rivers and groundwater.

• Increase your intake of chlorophyll (found in all green vegetables) and selenium (a trace mineral found in Brazil nuts, seafood and poultry), as these help to neutralize heavy metals allowing the body to excrete them.

WHAT YOU CAN DO TO HELP

There is little you can do to improve the air quality you are exposed to outside your home, but inside it there are many ways to find natural alternatives to the artificial fragrances found in household products and in cosmetic perfumes. Here are my top tips for creating all-round cleaner air.

• Buy ecologically friendly household cleaners, which contain only natural ingredients that do not release harmful fragrances.

• Open your windows often to refresh the air, rather than using aerosol sprays.

• Instead of chemical air fresheners, use aromatherapy essential oils in an oil burner or room sprays that are based on aromatherapy oils. Check the ingredients' labels carefully before you buy and choose products containing only natural rather than chemical ingredients.

- Replace regular scented candles with non-petroleum, vegetable wax varieties that use essential oils for their fragrance and not synthetic perfumes.
- Install hardwood or stone flooring instead of carpets, which harbour germs and are usually treated with fire-safe chemicals.
- Most people wear cosmetic perfume without even thinking of its effects, but I have seen severe reactions to perfumes – some reactions even altering moods. Remember that you put these fragrances on your skin and breathe them in all day long, so use a perfume that contains only essential oils. Be prepared to do some digging on this – many perfume companies will claim their ingredients are natural, but that does not necessarily mean the product contains essential oils alone. Ask your retailer to explain anything you don't understand on the label and work according to the general principle that most companies who do use only oils will be proud to say so on their packaging.

THE WATER YOU DRINK

Water is the body's second-most important nutrient after air, and on average it makes up around seventy percent of a person's body weight. Your body uses water for many purposes, including to lubricate your joints, to regulate your temperature, to protect your organs, to hydrate your cells, and to speed the elimination process by preventing constipation and encouraging your kidneys to flush out toxins in the urine.

Although tapwater is deemed safe to drink, many of our waterways may have been exposed to industrial, agricultural and pharmaceutical waste. Chemicals such as chlorine, as well as pesticides, herbicides and heavy metals, can leach into the soil and from there into our water sources. Another potential problem with tapwater is the level of hormones that may be in it. Hormone residues in the water – not only from pharmaceutical waste, but also from human waste as more and more women take Hormone Replacement Therapy and the contraceptive pill – may cause disturbing hormone imbalances in both men and women.

WHAT YOU CAN DO TO HELP

There are all sorts of ways to ensure the water you drink and use for cooking is as safe as it can be. Here are two of the most useful.

• Invest in a good-quality jug (pitcher) filter for water to use in hot drinks and for cooking, and consider having a permanent filter plumbed into your sink or tap. Sources indicate that most filters will eliminate a large proportion of the chemical residues in tapwater, including chlorine by-products and some insecticides and pesticides. Remember that even "permanent" filters need to be changed regularly (usually every six months) to keep their protection at optimum levels.

• Change to drinking bottled water that has been sourced from organic fields and that has a low sodium (salt) content. Choose water that is packaged in glass bottles instead of plastic, as chemicals in plastic can leach into the water, resulting in increased toxicity (especially hormone imbalance, as plastics may be manufactured with estrogen-like substances).

THE FOOD YOU EAT

As most of you will already know, much of the food available to you is preserved, flavoured and coloured artificially. The idea is that in these ways you can benefit from food that lasts longer, tastes better and looks prettier. However, the story is not ever that simple. Take meat, for example. In order to produce fleshy meat quickly, meat farmers may routinely give their animals antibiotics and growth hormones. While a cow grazes in a field, it may eat grass that itself is sprayed with pesticides, growth hormones and fertilizer, which in turn contaminate not only the cow's meat, but also its milk. Worst of all, while they are growing, fruit and vegetables are often sprayed up to 16 times with different toxic pesticides and fertilizers. Some of the chemicals in these products are so toxic to the human system that consumer pressure groups throughout the world are campaigning to ban them.

According to a report by the international organization Pesticide Action Network, which works with groups in more than ninety countries to try to minimize the use of chemicals on our food, more than five percent of fruit, vegetables and other foods carry harmful pesticide residues that pose "appreciable" health risks to consumers.

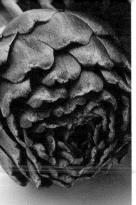

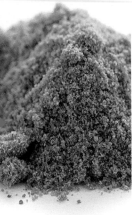

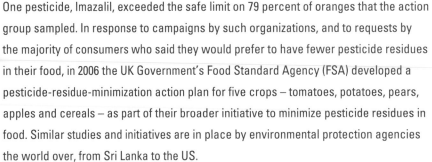

One pesticide, Imazalil, exceeded the safe limit on 79 percent of oranges that the action group sampled. In response to campaigns by such organizations, and to requests by the majority of consumers who said they would prefer to have fewer pesticide residues in their food, in 2006 the UK Government's Food Standard Agency (FSA) developed a pesticide-residue-minimization action plan for five crops – tomatoes, potatoes, pears, apples and cereals – as part of their broader initiative to minimize pesticide residues in food. Similar studies and initiatives are in place by environmental protection agencies the world over, from Sri Lanka to the US.

But the really great news is that we all have the ability to reduce our exposure to food toxins simply by changing some of our modern-day habits. So many of us now add to the toxic load on our body through our food because we have busy, stressful lives that leave us little time to spend making fresh food in the kitchen. We often welcome meals that we can prepare in an instant – but it's worth checking ourselves every now and then. As you reach for the instant micro-meal, try to remember how processing often strips packaged food of its nutritional value, how packaging itself (particularly in plastic; see p.33) may contaminate it, and how preservatives may increase its toxicity. Instead, follow a few simple steps that still make life easier – but, above all, make it healthier for you and anyone you might be cooking for.

WHAT YOU CAN DO TO HELP

The most important step any of us can take toward improving the food we eat is to buy only organic produce to cook with at home, and to eat organic as much as possible when we eat out. Although I believe that supplementation is necessary to optimize nutrient intake, research proves that organically grown food is higher in natural nutrients than non-organically grown food so, on the path to optimum health, I also firmly believe the organic route is essential. Once you've made the decision to switch to organic (and I promise you, you won't look back), follow these guidelines.

• Read every label before you buy. Look for preservatives and artificial colourants and flavourings on packets of food – and avoid them!

• Cook your own food from fresh, organic ingredients at home. If you have to have something at home that's non-organic, make sure you wash it thoroughly. (If you're short on time on weekdays, make batches of food over the weekends and freeze them so you at least have home-made fast food for during the week.) If you can, sign up for an organic box scheme or community-supported agriculture program (CSA). Not only will this bring organic ingredients to your door (with the added benefit of spending less time in the supermarket), it will also help you to eat foods that are fresh and seasonal.

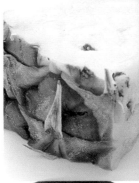

- Don't venture down the processed and ready-made food aisles in your supermarket.
- Say no to refined sugar – avoid pastries, cakes, cookies and so on; the same goes for artificial sugar. All kinds of sugar can cause highs and lows of energy way beyond the normal range, and this interferes with the proper functioning of your body.
- Drink juice or water, and avoid carbonated drinks – even the diet variety – as these contain high amounts of sugar (see above) and chemicals.

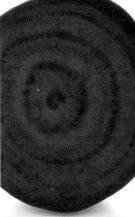

- Cut back on, or ideally eliminate completely, tea and coffee. Caffeine is your body's enemy, disrupting your energy levels and depleting your body of precious water. Processed, dried coffee is also full of additives and preservatives. Start the day with a glass of hot water with lemon and try different organic herbal teas instead (and remember that regular tea contains caffeine, too). If you must drink tea or coffee, choose organic, good-quality varieties and drink no more than two cups a day.
- Choose only the best organic wine, but try to avoid having more than a glass a day. Studies show that the tannins in red wine can be good for your circulation, but alcohol in any form is not, so the general rule has to be to drink only in moderation, and if you are doing a detox, cut out the wine completely.

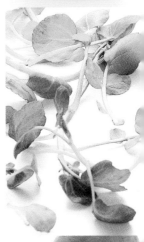

- Avoid all hydrogenated (trans) fats, which numerous studies show can raise your blood cholesterol levels. Although, if you eat organic, this guideline should follow naturally: hydrogenated fats are prohibited in the rules of organic status.

HOW TO EAT

It's not just what you eat, but how you eat it that affects your well-being. For example, it is essential to chew every mouthful and to mix it thoroughly with saliva, which contains digestive enzymes designed to relieve pressure on the digestive system. To get your saliva glands working, you need to appreciate what you're eating. Don't rush your meal, eat consciously and enjoy every mouthful.

five simple rules for eating well

Rule one: throw out your calorie counter Eating healthily is not about quantity, but about quality. You will find that you naturally eat the right balance of food if the food that you prepare and eat is made from fresh, preservative-free ingredients and you listen to your body when it tells you you've had enough.

Rule two: explore the world of food Choose a varied diet that does not involve the same foods repeatedly, as this can lead to food intolerance.

Rule three: attune to the seasons Select seasonal foods that are grown locally, where available. Apart from the fact that these foods will be the most fresh, seasonal eating will help you to avoid eating the same foods month in, month out.

Rule four: eat well Choose good-quality foods and, as much as possible, try to not be led by price. At least choose the best-quality organic produce you can afford.

Rule five: eat natural Prepare foods simply and naturally. Cook all your foods from fresh; bake or grill (broil) meats and fish; and lightly steam your vegetables. In these ways you can preserve much of the nutritional value of your food. When you can, eat foods raw – cruditées of carrot and celery with a homemade organic hummus dip is a delicious, healthy snack. And as much as possible, avoid microwaving, frying and roasting (which increase the action of free radicals in the body; see p.195), and steer clear of rich sauces, which your body finds hard to digest.

Stress greatly affects digestion, so it is also important to have quiet time to eat, in a peaceful environment ideally at a table. Make every mouthful small and put your knife and fork down between each one – this will help your brain to think your stomach is full, and prevent you from overeating. Don't feel guilty about leaving food on your plate if you've had enough. When you've finished, rest for five to ten minutes to let your food go down. Finally, try not to eat later than 8.30pm, so that your body gets enough time to digest your food before you go to bed (if your body is still digesting by bedtime, you will find it harder to sleep well).

a perfectly balanced diet

This pie chart represents the perfect diet. Most of your diet should comprise carbohydrates, which consist of whole grains (four servings a day, and include such foods as brown rice, millet, rye, oats, wholegrain bread and corn), vegetables (three servings a day), and fresh fruit (three servings a day). Try to divide the other thirty percent equally between fats (the equivalent of 1 tsp unsaturated oil, or 2 tbsp seeds) and protein (two servings per day). However, it's important that you eat "good" fats rather than bad, so keep saturated fat (from butter, meat and dairy) to a minimum and try instead to have your fat intake from unsaturated fats, such as cold-pressed vegetable oils (for example, olive oil) as well as from nuts and seeds (including sesame, walnut, sunflower, linseed/flax or pumpkin) and fish oils. Protein servings can come from eggs, quinoa, fish, beans or lentils, dairy or a small serving of meat.

fats

protein

carbohydrates

THE COSMETICS AND MEDICATIONS YOU USE

Although the idea that we ingest toxins from air, water and food is fairly well known, we rarely think about beauty and health products – cosmetics and medication – as culprits in toxicity. However, many cosmetics, for example, contain a common group of preservatives called parabens. These mimic the effects of the hormone estrogen in the body and have been named as a contributing cause of breast cancer. Other additives in cosmetics can cause headaches and mood swings, as well as being triggers for asthma and eczema. Most conventional medicines are made up of a cocktail of chemicals that can have adverse effects on the body. For example, some anti-inflammatory drugs for pain control were found to cause heart disease and were removed from the market. One of the most harmful chemical additives is malathion, which is often found in conventional treatment lotions for head lice. This insecticide can cause kidney, lung or brain damage, intestinal disorders, nose bleeds and immune problems, among other things. If you have children, follow the advice on pages 176–177 for treating lice – this home-made treatment is a safe and effective alternative. The following are some other effective ways to reduce the toxicity of the beauty and health products you use.

WHAT YOU CAN DO TO HELP

- Buy organic skin-care products and make-up wherever possible, and make it a rule not to buy something that contains an ingredient you don't recognize or can't pronounce. Always read the label yourself – take no one else's word for it.
- Remember that prevention is better than cure. Seek a homeopath or alternative health practitioner to work on improving your general health and to boost your immunity.

THE BODY'S OWN TOXINS

Most of us are unaware of this final group of toxins – the toxins the body produces itself. These toxins are by-products of the various aspects of metabolism that the body undertakes every day – including protein digestion, respiration and the breakdown of hormones in the liver. Also, bacteria and yeast, which are present in the gut, can generate toxic compounds. If you do not have sufficient bowel movements (that is, if you are constipated), these toxins may be absorbed back into the bloodstream and can damage the gut wall, leading to complaints such as leaky gut syndrome.

WHAT YOU CAN DO TO HELP

The following are three simple steps you can take to significantly reduce your body's self-imposed toxic load.

- Detox regularly – at least every three months. Regular detox not only helps the body to shed toxins that come from the outside, but also those that the body makes for itself.
- Help to prevent constipation and boost the movement of toxins out of your gut by

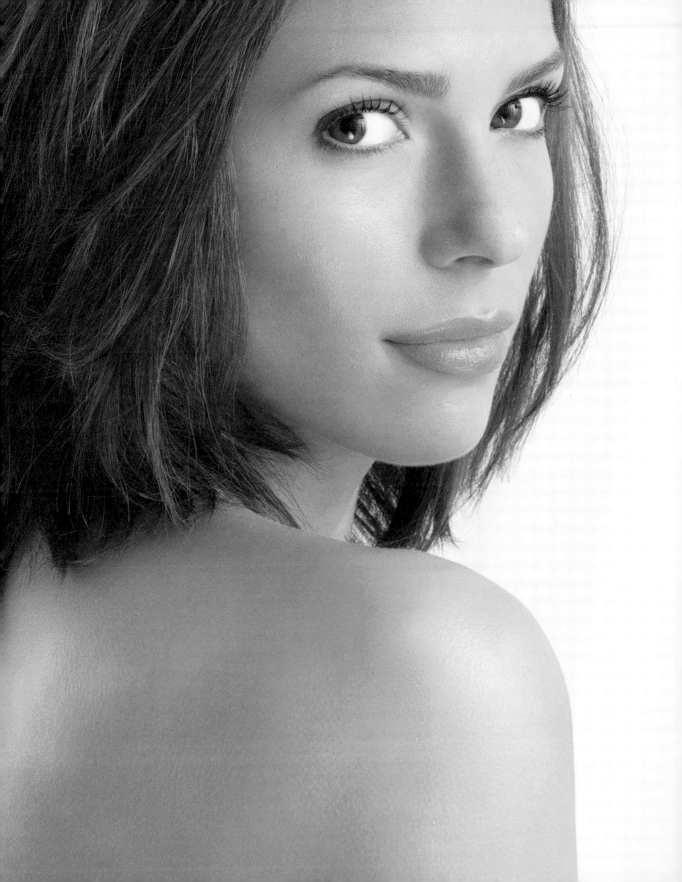

the natural first-aid kit

Another way to reduce your toxic load is to keep a natural first-aid kit for all the family. Ask a practitioner to make up the combinations for you.

For any injury Arnica, hypericum, rhus tox, ruta, symphytum and mag phos (Potency: 30c; two pillules, four times a day).

For fevers and earache Aconite, belladonna, chamomilla (Potency: 6c; ¼ tsp granules in a little water or straight into the mouth, up to six times a day).

For indigestion and bloating Lycopodium, carbo veg, nux vom (Potency: 6c; two pillules, three times a day).

For colds and flu Aconite, gelsemium, eupatorium, pyrogen, hepar sulph, ferrum phos (all at 6c potency) and anas barb (200c potency). (Two pillules, up to six times a day.)

For cuts and sore throats Hypericum, calendula and propolis tinctures in a combined spray applied directly to the cut or throat every hour if needed.

For bruising Arnica cream, applied four times a day to unbroken skin.

For skin infections Tea tree, manuka and neem cream, applied up to six times a day.

For burns Urtica and lavender cream, applied every hour for the first eight hours, then up to six times a day.

For food poisoning Arsenicum and mag phos (Potency: 6c or 30c; two pillules every 15 minutes, reducing to every hour, then three times a day as symptoms improve).

eating plenty of complex carbohydrates from whole grains, vegetables and fresh fruit, which are high in fibre. That's equivalent to three servings of vegetables, three servings of fruit and four servings of whole grains every day.

• Boost your diet with a probiotic supplement, which comprises some of the naturally occurring "good" bacteria your body needs to keep your digestive system in balance. The tangible results of this are that you should suffer less bloating and wind and feel generally that your immune system is working harder. Follow the dosage instructions on the packaging (or see my daily supplement plan on page 21).

the detox toolkit

A ten-day detox is the most important step you can take to beat back the toxins. In the course of your detox, you will see how you can make longlasting changes to your lifestyle to enable you to keep your health at its optimum levels. Over the following pages I will introduce you to the six essentials of a successful detox – they are my detox toolkit.

TOOL ONE: HEALTHY FOODS

The foods you eat during a detox should enhance the detox process, by supporting all the systems of elimination (see pp.28–29). Eat only organic produce that is seasonal and fresh, and free from preservatives and all artificial additives. Take a look at pages 33–35 for principles on how to choose healthy foods and follow these principles for the duration of your detox – and ideally beyond it.

TOOL TWO: CLEAN WATER

As we have already seen, like air, water is vital to life. It is worth reiterating here that both during a detox and as a general rule, it is important to drink only filtered tapwater, or bottled water from glass bottles and organic sources. You should drink at least eight glasses of water each day, between meals so as not to hamper digestion.

TOOL THREE: YOUR BREATH

When we take an in-breath, most of us use only the upper parts of our lungs. This is called shallow breathing. Breathing deeply, using the lower parts of the lungs, too, enables oxygen to circulate properly to your tissues, enriching them with nutrients and taking

my top twenty detox foods

The following is a list of 20 foods that I think are particularly brilliant at supporting the systems of elimination (especially the liver, kidneys and digestive system) during a detox. Antioxidants are also important during a detox as they help to rid the body of free radicals – unstable molecules that damage your body's cells (see p.195). Foods that are blood-cleansing act on the lymph, kidneys and skin to increase elimination via these routes. Before you begin your detox, stock your cupboards full of them and then enjoy using them in some delicious recipes. You will see they crop up lot in the recipes I've given during my ten-day detox (see pp.46–55), but by all means experiment with your own culinary creations.

Artichoke for the liver and
   bile-production

Turmeric for the liver; antioxidant

Rosemary for the circulation; antioxidant

Broccoli for the liver and bowel

Carrot for the liver and bowel

Celery for the kidneys; blood-cleansing

Fennel for the liver and kidneys;
   blood cleansing

Pineapple for the digestive system;
   anti-inflammatory

Papaya for the digestive system;
   cleansing

Beetroot (beet) for the liver

Radish for the liver

Watercress for the liver and bowel;
   blood-cleansing

Leeks for the liver, bowel and
   bile-production

Prunes for the bowel

Ginger for the digestion and circulation

Nuts and seeds for the bowel and liver

Cabbage for the liver and bowel

Green leafy vegetables for the liver

Apples for the liver and bowel

Pears for the liver and bowel

In addition, boost your intake of alfalfa sprouts (which are rich in the detox-boosting nutrients such as vitamins A and E, as well as the trace elements calcium, iron, potassium and phosphorous) and lemon, which helps to alkalize the body (see p.15).

waste away. Deep breathing also stimulates the lymphatic system (see p.29), a key part of immunity that helps to rid the body of toxins; and it induces a state of relaxation.

If you are unsure whether you breathe in a deep or shallow way, try this simple test. Stand or sit and place one hand on your solar plexus – which is found just below your ribcage – and the other on the lower abdomen. Breathe in and feel which hand moves. If it is your upper hand, you are shallow breathing; if the hand on your abdomen moves, you are deep breathing. Consciously breathe from the abdomen by taking in a deep breath so that your stomach rises and your lower hand moves; then breathe out. Do this for a few minutes until you get used to how it feels. Try to adopt deep breathing in normal life – check yourself from time to time, and make your breaths deeper if need be. Aim to change your breathing habits for the better, for ever.

TOOL FOUR: GENTLE EXERCISE

Exercise is vital for a healthy body and mind. However, during a detox program, it is important that you do not put undue stress on your body by undertaking a gruelling exercise regime. This would only divert energy away from the detoxification process and leave you feeling weakened. Instead, while you undertake the detox, switch to a more gentle and relaxing form of fitness, such as t'ai chi, yoga or walking. These forms of exercise are especially good for a detox because they encourage deep breathing, help to give your circulation a boost and encourage the flow of lymph. After any form of exercise it is important to stretch, as it releases the toxins that build up in the muscles during exercise. There are many excellent books on yoga and I recommend choosing a stretching sequence from one of these, or enlisting the help of a yoga teacher to find a suitable stretch for the end of your exercise program.

TOOL FIVE: MASSAGE

Like exercise, massage "moves" the body, increasing the circulation and improving oxygenation, and aiding the lymphatic system to help the removal of toxins from the tissues. On the first and third days of your detox, see a massage therapist for a full-body treatment lasting at least half an hour. On all the other detox days, try dry body-brushing (see p.44), which boosts the circulation and the flow of lymph, as well as

dry body-brushing

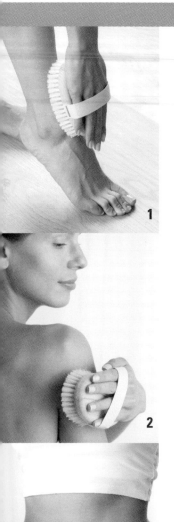

The best time to practise body-brushing is in the morning before you have a shower. Body brushes are available from most good beauty stores and pharmacies. Using counterclockwise movements, starting from the feet, brush the entire body, always working toward the heart to encourage the circulation of blood. Be gentle, so as not to make your skin red or sore. The whole practice should take no more than five minutes to complete.

1 Make sure that your body brush is completely clean, and then apply 4 drops neat rosemary essential oil to the brush. This is sufficient oil for the entire process. Starting with your right leg, place the body brush on the top of your right foot. Make small, very gentle, counterclockwise circular motions all over the foot (both on the top and underneath on the sole) before gradually moving all the way up your right leg. Then, make the same circular motions over the front and back of the leg. Repeat on your left foot and leg.

2 Now, starting at your right hand, make small, counterclockwise circular motions all over your hand and fingers and all the way up (both on the top and beneath) your right arm. Stop when you reach your right shoulder, then repeat on your left hand and arm as far as your shoulder.

3 Beginning on the lower left of your abdomen, make small, counterclockwise movements with the skin brush in a big counterclockwise circle around your belly button. When you reach the start again, move up your abdomen to your chest, always making circular movements, and brush the whole of your chest, moving across and upward until you reach your neck. When you have finished, rinse off the oil and dead skin cells with a warm shower.

having the added benefit of removing dead skin cells from the surface of the skin. (If you can't get to a therapist, use skin brushing every day.)

TOOL SIX: BALANCED MENTAL ENERGY

Most people with skin problems will tell you that their symptoms get worse during times of stress. This is principally because the body rechannels the energy required for detoxification to deal instead with anxiety. Negative emotions such as fear, self-pity and resentment have the same effect. I recommend two daily rituals to balance your mental energy during your detox. First, practise a daily meditation. Try a simple meditation on your breath. Find a quiet, calm place where you'll be undisturbed. Sit comfortably and breathe naturally for a few minutes, then close your eyes. Turn your focus to your breath. Breathe in deeply and, as you do so, in your head count slowly to five. Make the breath last the full count. Then, as you breathe out, count to five again. Continue breathing and counting in this way for as long as feels comfortable.

Second, a daily bath ritual (see below) provides an effective way to unwind at the end of the day to ensure a peaceful night's sleep that will allow your body to recharge and regenerate, making you better able to cope with stress and detoxification.

the detox bath ritual

This simple bath ritual is perfect for releasing stress at the end of the day and can also help to overcome insomnia. Practise it every day throughout your detox and at other times whenever you feel the need.

Fill the bath with comfortably warm water (not too hot) and add a few drops of a relaxing essential oil, such as lavender. Soak in the bath for 20 minutes. As you soak, close your eyes and run your mind over the day. Each time you come across a conversation, an incident or an issue that bothers you, imagine your anxiety about it flowing out of you and into the water. When you are ready to get out of the bath, pull out the plug and, as the water empties, imagine all your stresses swirling away, too.

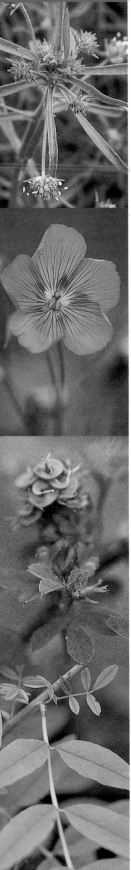

the ten-day detox

During the detox process your body will need support from a number of nutrients and herbs. An abundant supply of antioxidants, vitamins, fibre and essential fatty acids will enhance the process of cleansing and improve your body's ability to repair itself where toxins may have caused damage. In addition, there are several herbs that can actively speed up the detox process. The full detox program, which is outlined on pages 50–53, has been carefully compiled to contain everything your body needs to detoxify effectively. Follow my guidelines for detox and, far from depriving your body of anything, you will be giving your body a wealth of nutrients, as well as the tools to ensure a stress-free cleanse.

CLEANSING THE GUT

The starting point for your detox is to cleanse and repair your gut. As well as enabling nutrients to enter the blood more efficiently, a clean, restored gut means that your body's energy can focus on improving health in all your other systems, including the immune and nervous systems, to boost your overall well-being. Improvements to your circulation help to make your skin feel firmer and to reduce the appearance of age spots, pigmentation and wrinkles – they may even disappear. Best of all, a clean gut means that your energy will increase, making you feel rejuvenated and more able to cope with the life's demands.

GUT-CLEANSING HERBS AND OTHER REMEDIES

At The Organic Pharmacy we have a special mixture of the following natural remedies to support your detox. This mixture is available in capsule form and is called The Detox Colon Cleanse and Gut Repair. All our products are available in our shops or online.

PSYLLIUM HUSK This gentle but thorough intestinal cleanser relieves the autotoxemia (self-poisoning) that is caused by the growth of bacteria and fungi in the gut. Psyllium also helps to relieve constipation, a common cause of toxicity.

LINSEED Also known as flax seed, linseed helps to eliminate toxic waste in the bowels, improves blood-flow, and reduces inflammation in all the body's cells.

GREEN BARLEY This is a "perfect" food because it contains all the nutrients and amino acids the body requires to repair and rebuild cells, in a highly digestible form. Green barley contains chlorophyll, which gives green plants their colour and helps in particular to cleanse heavy metals (see box, p.31) from inside the gut.

CLAY Highly absorbent clay binds to impurities and heavy metals in the gut allowing them to be flushed out of the system.

ALFALFA This herb is a potent detoxifier, tonic and anti-inflammatory.

LICORICE This herb supports adrenal function (to regulate your hormones and energy levels) and has diuretic and laxative properties, which help to flush toxins from the system. Licorice also supports the liver (a primary organ of detoxification; see p.28), aids digestion and helps to repair gut damage.

L-GLUTAMINE This amino acid (a compound that forms the building blocks of proteins) plays a vital role in repairing the lining and mucous membranes of the gut.

ALOE VERA This super-strong species of aloe is well known for its cleansing and repairing properties. It is one of my star ingredients (see pp.106–107).

GINGER A well-known anti-inflammatory, ginger improves the circulation and digestion and can soothe intestinal cramps. It can also cleanse and repair the gut.

herbal detox support drops

While the body is going through the detox process, it is absolutely vital to support the organs of elimination in as many ways as possible. So, as well as the remedies on this page, use a mixture of equal measures of the following herbal tinctures (make sure they are made using organic ingredients), which a qualified herbalist or pharmacist can make up for you. All the herbs in this combination help to support your liver and kidneys. Take 15 drops of the combined tinctures in a little water three times a day during your detox.

• milk thistle • dandelion • red clover • artichoke • turmeric • berberis • marsh mallow

NUTRIENT SUPPORT

When detoxifying, your body needs a ready source of antioxidants, phytonutrients, essential fats and B-vitamins to give your organs the fuel they need to cleanse your body as quickly as possible. Furthermore, during the detoxification process, the body releases more free radicals (atoms that damage cells; see p.195) than normal, which makes proper nutrient support in the form of supplementation essential.

SUPPLEMENTS TO SUPPORT YOUR DETOX

The following may seem like a lot of supplements, but I thoroughly recommend taking them individually (rather than in a combined supplement) during your ten-day detox – after all, it's only for a short time and your body will thank you. (Return to your usual supplement regime after the ten days.) I have given guidelines on dosages, but each brand will be different, so check the packet instructions, too.

ANTIOXIDANTS You need antioxidants to mop up free radicals, maintain skin integrity and promote healing. Look for capsules that contain at least vitamin (ester) C, vitamin E, pycnogenol (pine bark extract) and green tea.
DOSAGE Two capsules with lunch and two with dinner, daily.
MULTI-VITAMINS Your body will absorb and process plant-based supplements much more easily than any other, so look for multi-vitamins containing plant foods such as spirulina, alfalfa, wheatgrass, barley grass, blue green algae, broccoli, carrot, blueberry, bilberry, grapeskin and cranberry.
DOSAGE Two capsules with lunch and two with dinner, daily.
ESSENTIAL FATTY ACIDS (EFAs) These are important during detox because they help the body with the process of cell renewal. Look for EFA supplements that contain the following co-factors, which will help to ensure your body absorbs the essential fats properly: lecithin (to emulsify fats and support the liver); phosphatydyl choline, inositol and choline (to help to stabilize cell membranes and regenerate liver cells); and linseed (flax seed), evening primrose and borage (to improve mood, hormone balance, and skin and gut health).
DOSAGE Two capsules each morning.

B-COMPLEX VITAMINS During a detox pimples may break out on the surface of your skin. This is all part of the cleansing process and shouldn't alarm you. Nevertheless, B-vitamins help to speed healing in pimples, as well as to combat any stress.
DOSAGE One capsule each morning.

MAGNESIUM AND CALCIUM This combined supplement is important for maintaining the nervous system, easing the muscles and aiding sleep during the detox.
DOSAGE 1,000mg half an hour before bed, every day.

PROBIOTICS These provide "friendly" bacteria and your body needs them in abundance during a detox.
DOSAGE Two billion, twice a day.

YOUR STEP-BY-STEP TEN-DAY DETOX PROGRAM

Before you begin your detox, fill your cupboards and refrigerator with my top detox foods and the other foods mentioned in my recommended daily menu plans (see pp.50–53). Stock up on the recommended herbs and supplements and any items you'll need for body treatments to support you through the detoxification process.

The first three days of the program are the hardest, so if you work conventional hours, start your detox on a Friday morning and try to plan as little as possible for that day and the coming weekend. Remember that you need lots of energy for detoxification, so rest is vital. If you feel tired, sleep.

EVERY DAY

• On waking, drink a glass of hot water with half a lemon squeezed in it. This helps to break down mucus in the body and alkalizes your tissues (see p.15).

• Take three herbal detox capsules (see p.46–47) with a full glass of water twice a day – half an hour before a meal or one hour after a meal is best.

• Do ten minutes of breathing exercises followed by ten minutes of stretching (see p.43). If time is tight, reduce this to five minutes of each.

• Before showering, gently dry brush the skin (see p.44).

• Shower and massage the body with body oil containing rosemary and grapefruit essential oils, to boost your circulation.

step-by-step detox:
days one to five

DAY ONE

BREAKFAST: Blend ½ mango, 1 banana and 230ml/8fl oz/1 scant cup low-fat plain bio yogurt.

MID-MORNING SNACK: 1 apple or 1 pear.

LUNCH: Chickpea and Quinoa Salad. Cook 200g/7oz/1 cup quinoa, as directed on the packet, then add 100g/3½oz/½ cup drained, canned chickpeas, 1 chopped carrot, 1 tbsp extra-virgin olive oil and 1 large handful chopped parsley leaves. You can make this the night before and store it in the fridge. (Serves 1.)

MID-AFTERNOON SNACK: A handful of nuts or seeds.

DINNER: Revitalizing and Immune-boosting Soup (p.54)

DAY TWO

BREAKFAST: 2 slices walnut bread with honey and a cup of green tea.

MID-MORNING SNACK: 2 prunes.

LUNCH: Celery Soup with a slice of spelt bread. Heat 1 tbsp olive oil in a wok, add ½ chopped onion, 1 chopped carrot, 1 chopped celery stick and 1 leek, white part chopped. Stir-fry until soft. Add 625ml/21½fl oz/2½ cups vegetable bouillon and 100g/3½oz/1 cup pearl barley; cook for 45 minutes, until the barley is soft. Add 1 tbsp each chopped thyme leaves and 1 tbsp chopped rosemary leaves and serve. (Serves 2.)

MID-AFTERNOON SNACK: A glass of Detox Juice (see box, p.53).

DINNER: Nourishing Carrot Soup (p.54).

DAY THREE

BREAKFAST: 2 eggs – poached, soft-boiled or scrambled.

MID-MORNING SNACK: A handful of grapes.

LUNCH: Chicken Soup. Place 1 chopped fennel bulb, 1 sprig thyme, chopped, the juice of ½ lemon, 1 leek, white part chopped, and 30g/1oz/¼ cup broccoli florets in a large saucepan and pour in 750ml/26fl oz/3 cups organic chicken stock. Bring to a boil and leave to simmer for 1 hour. You can prepare this the night before and leave it in the fridge overnight. (Serves 4.)

MID-AFTERNOON SNACK: A glass of Detox Juice (see box, p.53).

DINNER: Cream Wörthersee Spread (p.54) on 2 or 3 slices of wholegrain wheat, rye or spelt bread, or sourdough.

DAY FOUR

BREAKFAST: Small bowl of unsweetened muesli with skimmed milk.

MID-MORNING SNACK: 1 or 2 unsalted, plain rice cakes.

LUNCH: Watercress, Avocado and Alfalfa Pitta (below). Mix together 25g/1oz watercress, ½ chopped avocado and 25g/1oz alfalfa sprouts. Whisk together 2 tbsp low-fat plain bio yogurt, 1 tbsp olive oil, juice of ½ lemon and 1 tsp smooth mustard. Season lightly with sea salt and pour over the salad mixture. Place in a wholegrain pitta and serve.

MID-AFTERNOON SNACK: 1 pear.

DINNER: Mixed Vegetable Quinoa (see p.55).

DAY FIVE

BREAKFAST: 1 cupful of chopped fresh fruit, served with 250g/9oz/1 cup low-fat plain bio yogurt.

MID-MORNING SNACK: A handful of cucumber and carrot sticks.

LUNCH: Mint and Feta Salad (p.55).

MID-AFTERNOON SNACK: A handful of nuts or seeds.

DINNER: Grilled Chicken Thighs. Remove the skin from 2 chicken thighs and grill (broil) under a medium-hot grill (broiler) for 4 minutes each side until cooked through. Steam 2 or 3 chopped carrots and 150g/5½oz/1 cup peas, for 2–3 minutes until tender. Sprinkle with 1 tbsp chopped parsley or mint and serve either warm or cold. (Serves 2.)

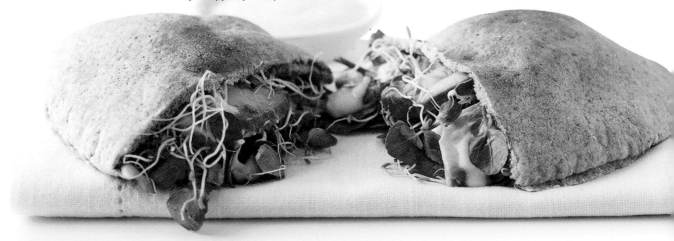

step-by-step detox: days six to ten

DAY SIX

BREAKFAST: 5 or 6 mushrooms sautéed in olive oil and served on rye toast.

MID-MORNING SNACK: A piece of fruit of your choice.

LUNCH: 3 plain, unsalted rice cakes with 50g/2oz/¼ cup hummus and 3 or 4 cherry tomatoes.

MID-AFTERNOON SNACK: A handful of carrot and cucumber sticks.

DINNER: Revitalizing and Immune-boosting Soup (p.54) with Cream Wörthersee Spread (p.54) on 2 or 3 slices of wholegrain wheat, rye or spelt bread, or sourdough.

DAY SEVEN

BREAKFAST: 2 pieces fruit (your choice), chopped, and served with 2 tbsp low-fat plain bio yogurt.

MID-MORNING SNACK: A piece of fruit of your choice.

LUNCH: Avocado Pitta. Mix together ½ chopped avocado, 25g/1oz alfalfa sprouts and 1 Little Gem lettuce or heart of Romaine, shredded, drizzle with olive oil and lemon juice and place in a wholemeal pitta bread.

MID-AFTERNOON SNACK: A handful of nuts and seeds.

DINNER: Vegetable and Chickpea Couscous (follow the recipe for vegetable and quinoa salad from Day One, substituting couscous for the quinoa).

DAY EIGHT

BREAKFAST: Pineapple, Papaya and Mango smoothie. Blend 5 large chunks pineapple, ½ chopped papaya and ½ chopped mango and 250ml/9fl oz/1 cup low-fat plain bio yogurt.

MID-MORNING SNACK: One oatcake with low-fat cream cheese.

LUNCH: Vegetable Quinoa. Place 50g/2oz/¼ cup quinoa in a saucepan with 2 chopped celery sticks, 1 chopped fennel bulb, 1 leek, white part chopped, and 1 chopped carrot. Pour in 150ml/5fl oz/scant ⅔ cup vegetable stock and 1 tbsp extra-virgin olive oil, bring to the boil, cover and leave to simmer for 10 minutes until the quinoa is soft, then serve. (Serves 1.)

MID-AFTERNOON SNACK: A piece of fruit of your choice.

DINNER: Prawn and Vegetable Stir-Fry (below). Gently heat 1 tbsp coconut or olive oil in a wok, add 1 crushed clove garlic, 1cm/½in piece root ginger, finely chopped, and ½ deseeded, finely chopped red chili and stir-fry. Add 2 spring onions (scallions), white part chopped, 75g/2½oz mangetout (snow peas), 100g/4oz chopped pak choi, and 5 chopped shiitake mushrooms. Stir-fry for 5 minutes, then add 6 raw, peeled king prawns. Fry for 5 minutes more, until the prawns are cooked. Stir in a squeeze of lime juice and serve immediately on a handful baby spinach leaves. (Serves 1.)

DAY NINE

BREAKFAST: Small bowl of unsweetened muesli with skimmed milk.

MID-MORNING SNACK: 1 oatcake with low-fat cream cheese.

LUNCH: Nourishing Carrot Soup (p.54).

MID-AFTERNOON SNACK: A piece of fruit of your choice.

DINNER: Mixed Vegetable Quinoa (p.55).

DAY TEN

BREAKFAST: 2 eggs – poached, soft-boiled or scrambled.

MID-MORNING SNACK: 2 prunes.

LUNCH: Mint and Feta Salad (p.55).

MID-AFTERNOON SNACK: A glass of Detox Juice (see box, right).

DINNER: Mixed Vegetable Quinoa (p.55).

detox juice

Blend the juice of ¼ beetroot (beet), ½ lemon, 2 celery sticks and 2 carrots with a pinch of turmeric and ½ tsp extra-virgin olive oil.

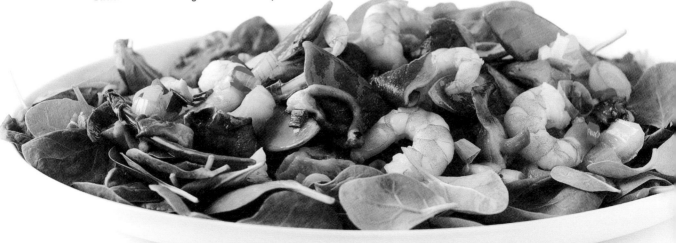

my five must-have detox recipes

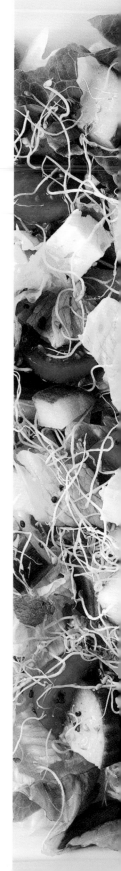

Revitalizing and Immune-boosting Soup

Serves 4

1 litre/35fl oz/4 cups vegetable stock

100g/4oz/½ cup brown rice or

50g/2oz/¼ cup pearl barley (optional)

6 shiitake mushrooms, chopped

1 spring onion (scallion), white part sliced

1cm/½in piece root ginger, finely chopped

½ red chili, deseeded and finely chopped, or ¼ tsp dried red chili

2 sprigs thyme, leaves chopped

2 carrots, finely diced

If using the barley or rice, place in a large saucepan and add the stock. Bring to the boil and leave to simmer for 20 minutes. Add the remaining ingredients and continue to simmer for a further 10 minutes. If not using them, place all the ingredients in a large saucepan, bring to the boil and leave to simmer for 10 minutes. Season to taste and serve with a squeeze of lime or lemon.

Nourishing Carrot Soup

Serves 4

100g/4oz floury potatoes or 1 sweet potato, finely diced

150g/6oz baby carrots, diced

1 litre/35fl oz/4 cups vegetable stock

1 tbsp low-fat sour cream

1 tbsp finely chopped nettles, watercress or parsley

a little grated nutmeg

Place the potatoes, carrots and stock in a large saucepan, bring to the boil and leave to simmer until soft. Pour 1 tablespoon of the liquid into the sour cream and stir until smooth. Pour the sour cream mixture back into the rest of the soup, add half of the nettles, watercress or parsley and the nutmeg, and blend. Sprinkle the remaining herbs on top and serve. For a thicker soup use a little less liquid or a few more vegetables.

Cream Wörthersee Spread

Serves 4

250g/9oz/1 cup cottage cheese

1 tbsp chervil, finely chopped

4 tbsp cow's, sheep's or goat's milk

½ beetroot (beet) or 2 carrots diced and cooked or 180g/6½oz raw spinach cooked and chopped

sea salt

Mix together all the ingredients to make a chunky spread. You can substitute silken tofu for the cottage cheese and oat, rice or soy milk for the cow's, sheep's or goat's milk, if you prefer.

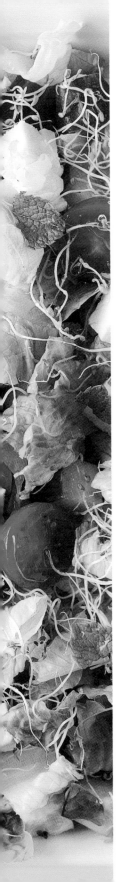

Mixed Vegetable Quinoa

300cl/11fl oz/2 cups vegetable stock

100g/3½oz/½ cup quinoa

1 tbsp olive oil

1 celery stick, chopped

2 spring onions (scallions), white part chopped

1 sweet potato, chopped

1 courgette (zucchini), chopped

50g/2oz/½ cup broccoli florets

1 large handful chopped parsley

Serves 2

Place the stock and quinoa in a large saucepan, bring to the boil and leave to simmer for 7–8 minutes. In a heavy-bottomed pan, heat the olive oil and fry the celery, spring onions and sweet potato over a low heat for 2–3 minutes. Add the courgette and broccoli and continue to fry for 3 minutes. Stir the vegetables into the quinoa mixture and simmer until all the liquid is absorbed. Sprinkle with the parsley, and lemon if desired, and serve.

Mint and Feta Salad (left)

1 tbsp olive oil

1 tbsp apple cider vinegar

1 head Romaine lettuce, chopped

handful alfalfa sprouts

4 sprigs mint, leaves chopped

5 cherry tomatoes, halved

½ cucumber, chopped

8 small cubes feta cheese

sea salt

Serves 2

In a small bowl, whisk together the oil and vinegar. Mix together all the remaining ingredients in a large bowl, drizzle the dressing over the salad and season with salt. Serve either on its own or with a small portion of grilled (broiled) or steamed lamb or chicken.

my favourite detox smoothies

Detox Antioxidant Smoothie

• 5 blueberries • 5 strawberries

• 5 goji berries (optional) • 1 kiwi • ½ lemon or 1 tbsp apple cider vinegar

Put all the ingredients and 3 tbsp water in a blender and whiz until smooth. Serve as a breakfast or mid-morning snack.

Digestive Enzyme Smoothie

• 2 slices pineapple • ½ papaya, cubed

• 2 tbsp low-fat plain bio yogurt

• ½ lemon (optional) • 1 sprig mint

Put all the ingredients in a blender and whiz until smooth. Enjoy after any meal to help your digestive system in its important work.

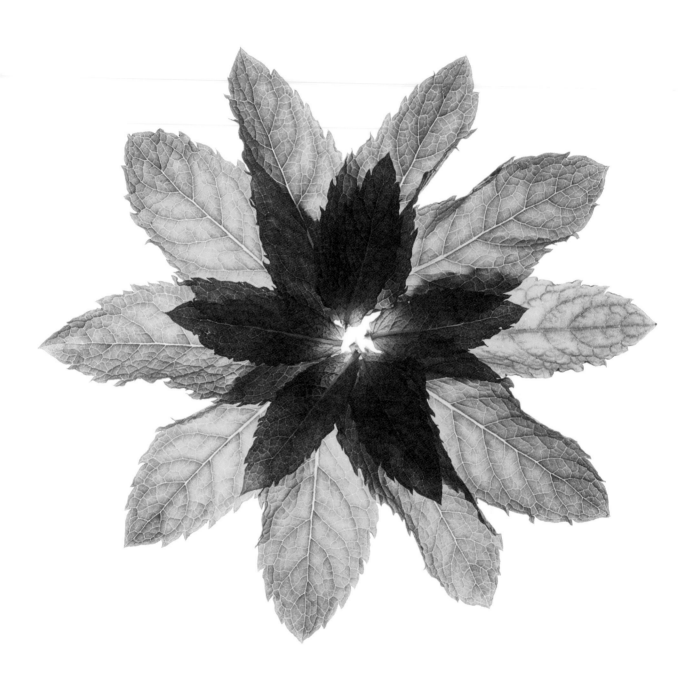

CHAPTER 2

healing common complaints

In order for you to be healthy and feel full of vitality, your body needs to be in a state of balance. When its systems are over- or under-stimulated, your health will suffer. Thankfully, your amazing body has been designed with an immune system that usually enables it to heal itself. Sometimes, however, this remarkable capacity for self-healing is diminished, especially when the root cause of an illness is relentless – for example, when the body suffers endless stress or a poor diet, or is over-exposed to toxins.

Identifying the causes of imbalance and eliminating them (such as by finding time to relax, eating healthily and reducing the toxic load) are first steps to long-term health, well-being and beauty. Then, when illness does hit, my three-pronged approach to treatment, using herbs, supplements and homeopathic remedies, can kickstart – and even speed up – the healing process. This chapter features the 12 health complaints that we are most commonly asked to treat at The Organic Pharmacy. For each ailment I have given you step-by-step advice on which wonderful herbs, supplements and homeopathic remedies will encourage self-healing so that your body can use its own defence mechanisms to fight that particular illness and bring its systems back into balance.

left: peppermint (*Mentha piperita*)

bacterial and viral infections

Bacteria and viruses surround us. A healthy immune system is generally able to fight off these pathogens, but many factors in our environment (including stress, overwork and toxicity), coupled with a poor diet high in sugars and additives and low in nutrients, compromise immunity, making us susceptible to illness.

The Treatment Program

Herbs, supplements and homeopathic remedies provide an arsenal of immune-boosters, as well as antibacterials and antivirals, to assist the body's recovery from infection. Although many of the conditions in the rest of this chapter also fall under the umbrella of "bacterial and viral infections", this treatment program provides a useful cure-all.

RECOMMENDED HERBS

The following are the herbs I have found give optimum results for boosting immunity against infection. When the first symptoms of illness appear, take 15 drops of each tincture in a little water or juice at least three times a day for the duration of your illness.

ASTRAGALUS (*Astragalus membranaceus*) This herb inhibits viruses and can destroy bacteria. It increases the body's production of immune-boosting white blood cells.

CAT'S CLAW (*Uncaria tomentosa*) Cat's claw contains compounds called pentacyclic oxindole alkaloids, which stimulate the body's production of immune cells.

ECHINACEA (*Echinacea purpurea*) Echinacea boosts production of the protein interferon (which helps to kill viruses) and of infection-fighting white blood cells. It contains alkylamides, which are thought to prevent bacteria penetrating the skin.

GOLDENSEAL (*Hydrastis canadensis*) Alkaloids in goldenseal increase the production of white blood cells and its astringency clears mucus.

THYME (*Thymus vulgaris*) Antiseptic and antimicrobial, thyme will generally help to clear the body of infection. It will promote restful sleep to speed recovery.

ELDERBERRY (*Sambucus nigra*) The berries of the elder tree contain antiviron, which

right: echinacea (*Echinacea purpurea*)

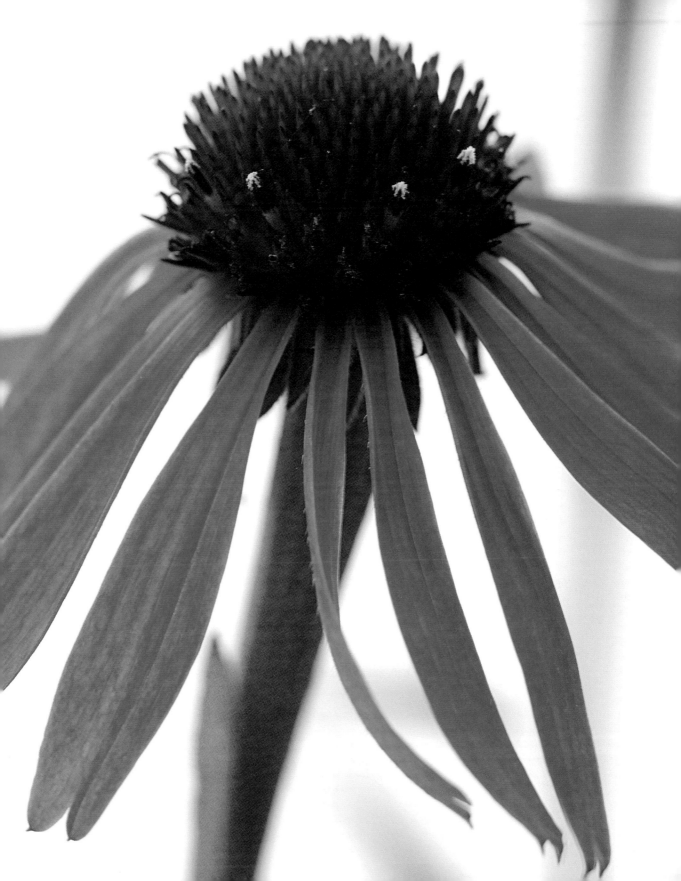

reduces viral symptoms, and antioxidant flavonoids to speed recovery.

PLANTAIN (*Plantago major*) Plantain contains anti-inflammatory and antibacterial properties. It is particularly useful for combatting gut and respiratory infections.

ST JOHN'S WORT (*Hypericum perforatum*) This excellent antiviral (see pp.138–139) is ideal for combatting colds, flu, and herpes infections.

OLIVE LEAF (*Olea europaea*) Olive leaf's main active constituent is oleuropein, a powerful antiviral that is thought to act by either destroying the virus's cell walls or inhibiting the production of enzymes and amino acids the virus needs to grow.

LEMON BALM (*Melissa officinalis*) Phenolic acid in lemon balm prevents a virus attaching itself to cells and so stops it spreading through the body.

ESSENTIAL SUPPLEMENTS

Take the following supplements when you feel or notice the first symptoms of infection, and continue taking them until you feel well again.

what is an infection?

Bacterial infections are caused by microscopic, single-celled organisms (bacteria) and include pneumococcal infections (such as sinusitis, meningitis and pneumonia) and staphylococcal infections (such as skin infections and food poisoning). A virus is much smaller than a bacterium. It invades a living cell to replicate, releasing new viruses before it eventually dies. The new viruses infect other cells, and so it goes on. Viral infections include the common cold, flu, shingles, herpes simplex (cold sores), and yellow fever. Your body becomes more susceptible to bacterial and viral infections when your immune system is weak. A poor diet lacking in nutrients (in particular, vitamins A, C and B-complex and the minerals zinc and selenium), as well as stress, high toxicity and over-reliance on medication or other drugs, all contribute to weakened immunity. In addition, a healthy gut contains good bacteria that stimulate lymph tissue in the gut wall. This tissue is responsible for producing antibodies against pathogens. So, an unhealthy digestive system can lead to infection, too.

ANTIOXIDANTS Crucial for preventing free radicals from damaging our cells, many antioxidants, such as vitamin (ester) C and zinc, possess immune-boosting properties.
DOSAGE Two capsules, twice a day.
PROBIOTICS These "good" bacteria provide a biological barrier to the invasion and establishment of pathological bacteria.
DOSAGE Eight billion daily during an infection.

RECOMMENDED HOMEOPATHIC REMEDIES

The following is a selection of the homeopathic remedies I have found to be most effective at fighting infections. Take them in a 6c or 30c potency, three times a day.

MERC SOL, THUJA, PULSATILLA This combination is excellent for infections that have a green, foul-smelling discharge from the nose or ears, or in the sputum.
HEPAR SULPH This remedy will help to push the infection out as pus, so it is great for boils or other topical infections.
PYROGENIUM, GELSEMIUM, EUPATORIUM This combination is excellent for flu-type infections with aching muscles.

NUTRITIONAL ADVICE

Always follow the general healthy-eating guidelines on pages 34–35 when trying to fight any infection, as well as adhering to the following recommendations.

FOODS TO EAT

Increase your intake of immune-boosters such as garlic, shiitake mushrooms, oranges and other fresh fruit, and all fresh vegetables, especially sweet potatoes. Thyme, cinnamon and garlic will provide antiseptic properties, while ginger will keep inflammation to a minimum. Stock up on the chicken soup, too (see p.69).

FOODS TO AVOID

Keep dairy products (except for plain bio yogurt and cottage cheese) to a minimum, as these tend to be mucus-forming so may make your symptoms worse.

colds and flu

A cold is a viral infection in the upper respiratory tract caused by any one of 120 viruses known as rhinoviruses. Flu (influenza) is also caused by a virus and has similar symptoms to a cold, but these tend to be more severe.

The Treatment Program

Cold symptoms include headaches, a sore throat, a cough, a running or blocked nose, sinus pain, and tiredness. Flu usually has all of these symptoms and also eye ache, glandular swelling, and melancholy. It is important to treat the cold or flu virus, but it is also vital to strengthen the immune system against the infection.

RECOMMENDED HERBS

Take a combination of any of the herbs listed on pages 58–60, such as thyme, at the first symptoms of a cold or the flu. Repeat this combination every one to two hours during the day, for at least two or three days. Reduce the frequency as symptoms improve.

ESSENTIAL SUPPLEMENTS

VITAMIN (ESTER) C Research shows that vitamin C helps to improve immunity by increasing the production of the virus-inhibitor interferon, as well as other immune cells.
DOSAGE 500mg, four times a day.
ZINC An antiviral and antioxidant, zinc is crucial for the proper function of immune cells.
DOSAGE 15mg, twice a day.
VITAMIN A By speeding the healing of the mucous membranes of the lungs and throat, vitamin A can help to combat catarrh and congestion.
DOSAGE One 5,000iu capsule, daily. (Avoid vitamin A if you are pregnant.)

RECOMMENDED HOMEOPATHIC REMEDIES

The symptoms of a cold or flu can change over the course of a week. Each stage needs its own remedy, so I have listed here the most appropriate remedies for the common

right: thyme (*Thymus vulgaris*)

phases of a cold. I recommend a 30c or 200c potency every two hours for the first 12 to 24 hours, and then three times a day until you have recovered.

ABC (aconite, belladonna, chamomilla) This is an excellent homeopathic combination both for adults and for children in the very first stages of infection.

COLD AND FLU MIXTURE (aconite, gelsemium, hepar sulph, pyrogen, eupatorium, anas barb) Take this mixture at the onset of cold symptoms, when you have aching, sore or heavy muscles; and at the beginning of a sore throat or fever.

SINUS AND CATARRH MIXTURE (pulsatilla, hepar sulph, merc sol, thuja, hydrastis, kali bich) This mixture is especially effective if you have green or yellow mucus, and during the latter stages of a cold or flu. (See also Coughs; p.76–79.)

NUTRITIONAL ADVICE

Eat the foods that help to overcome a cough (see p.79), and, in addition, eat nuts and seeds, which supply antioxidants and zinc. Avoid sugar, which inhibits immunity.

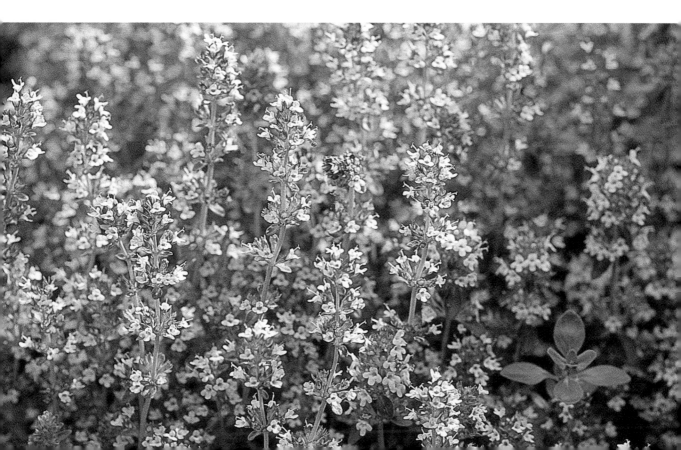

fever

One of the body's defence mechanisms, a fever is an elevated temperature (above 38°C/100°F), which not only increases the body's production of immune-fighting cells, but also makes the body a more hostile environment to bacteria and viruses.

The Treatment Program

Leave a fever alone unless it reaches above 40°C (104°F), when you risk seizure – in which case seek medical advice. Sweating is the body's way to cool down and any treatment program must include ways in which to encourage it.

RECOMMENDED HERBS

Take the following herbs at the first signs of fever. Unless otherwise stated, take the standard dosage of 15 drops of each tincture in water or juice, three times a day.

YARROW (*Achillea millefolium*) As well as helping to promote perspiration, the volatile oil in this herb has been shown to have anti-inflammatory properties.

PEPPERMINT (*Mentha piperita*) This wonderful herb stimulates the circulation, which promotes sweating and reduces fever. It is also a decongestant. Take it as an infusion.

treating childhood fevers

These remedies are safe for children over six months old, unless otherwise stated.

ABC At the first sign of symptoms, give one pill in a 30c or 200c potency every hour for the first three or four doses, then three times a day until symptoms have gone.

Immune-boosting tonic Give 5 drops of astragalus or elderberry tincture in a little water or juice up to five times a day for one week.

Vitamin (ester) C Give 250mg in juice twice a day for a week to children over age two.

To generally boost the immune system against the viral and bacterial infections that often cause a fever, also take the following herbs at the standard dosage:
• astragalus (see p.58) • echinacea (see p.58) • goldenseal (see p.58) • elderberry (p.58)

ESSENTIAL SUPPLEMENTS

There are no supplements that will specifically reduce a fever, but it is essential to take supplements that will boost your immune response. The two most important are:
• vitamin (ester) C (500mg, four times daily; see p.62) • zinc (15mg, twice daily; see p.62)

RECOMMENDED HOMEOPATHIC REMEDIES

The following remedies are best for fever. Take them in a 30c or 200c potency, five times a day from the first signs of fever. Stop taking them when the fever has abated.

ABC (aconite, belladonna, chamomilla) This is the number-one fever remedy. Combine ABC with ferrum phos (see below) at the first sign of a fever.
FERRUM PHOS Take this at the first sign of a fever. It is especially good if your fever is accompanied by pain on swallowing and aching in the back and limbs.
MERC SOL AND PULSATILLA This combination will speed recovery, especially when a fever is accompanied by earache or green mucus.

NUTRITIONAL ADVICE

If you have a fever, boost your intake of immunity foods and of anything that increases your circulation to make you sweat (see below). There's no need to avoid any specific foods, but do steer clear of dairy products, which are mucus-forming, and junk foods.

FOODS TO EAT

Garlic, thyme, cinnamon and citrus fruits are all good immune-boosters when you have a fever, while ginger provides anti-inflammatory properties as well as antibacterial properties to fight any infection. Ginger also helps to promote sweating, as does chili. I also recommend the Chicken Soup (see p.69).

sore throats

Anything that irritates and inflames the lining of the throat can cause soreness, and a sore throat is usually the result of any one of several different conditions. An inflammation of the throat itself is called pharyngitis; an inflammation of the voice box is called laryngitis; and an inflammation of the tonsils is called – yes, you guessed it! – tonsillitis. Most sore throats are the result of viral infections, usually as part of a cold or the flu (see pp.62–63), and you can usually treat these quickly and easily at home. However, a small percentage of sore throats come from bacterial infections – usually the streptococcus bacteria. The symptoms of streptococcal infection develop quickly and include a high fever with red, swollen tonsils and tender, sore lymph nodes at the sides of the throat. For children, especially, you should consult your doctor if you suspect a bacterial sore throat.

The Treatment Program

To give yourself the best chance of overcoming a sore throat quickly, treat it at the first signs of infection – as soon as you have that tender, crackling sensation that makes it uncomfortable to swallow. I have found the following remedy combinations to be extremely effective.

RECOMMENDED HERBS

Use the following herbal remedies either individually or in combination. The standard dosage is 15 drops of tincture (of each tincture, if you are combining remedies) in a little water or juice three times a day. Use this unless otherwise stated.

SAGE (*Salvia officinalis*) Wonderfully therapeutic, sage essential oil contains the compound salvene, which gives the oil both antibacterial and antiseptic actions. *DOSAGE* 10 drops tincture in a little water, three or four times a day.
CALENDULA (*Calendula officinalis*) One of my Star Ingredients, calendula (see pp.126–127), is a must-have for sore throats because of its strong antiseptic and

antibacterial properties. It also helps to soothe pain and reduce fever and inflammation. Use the standard dosage.

PROPOLIS (_Resina propoli_) Made by bees from tree sap, propolis is not strictly a herb, but medicinally it is used as such. Antiseptic, antibiotic, antibacterial, antifungal and antiviral, propolis is available as a tincture (take it at the standard dosage) and also as a ready-made throat spray. To use propolis as a gargle, add 5ml (1 tsp) propolis tincture to 100ml (3½fl oz) cooled, boiled water.

DOSAGE Gargle up to three times a day until symptoms subside. Swallow the gargle.

MYRRH (_Commiphora myrrha_) Another antiseptic and anti-inflammatory herb, myrrh makes a soothing gargle for acute sore throats. Place 5 drops myrrh tincture in 50ml (1½fl oz) cooled, boiled water and stir.

DOSAGE Gargle with the mixture up to six times a day (it will help if you swallow the gargle, too) until your symptoms subside, then reduce this to only three times a day until you have made a full recovery.

SUPPLEMENTARY HERBS

It's also important to boost the immune system against sore-throat infections, in which case you should use the following immune-friendly herbs at the standard dosage:
• astragalus (see p.58) • echinacea (see p.58) • elderberry (see p.58)

ESSENTIAL SUPPLEMENTS

Boost your intake of antivirals, antibacterials and antioxidants to help your body fight off the throat infection. Increase your dosages of the following supplements as indicated until symptoms subside:
• vitamin (ester) C (500mg, four times daily; see p.62) • zinc (15mg, twice daily; see p.62)

RECOMMENDED HOMEOPATHIC REMEDIES

Use the homeopathic remedies on the following page in combination as soon as your symptoms first appear. It will help to take all the remedies – even those that don't necessarily have an exact "match" for your symptoms (see p.16). Use a 6c or 30c potency of each remedy, six times a day.

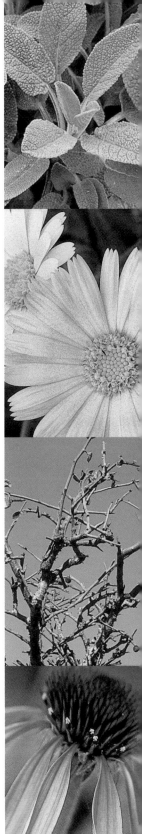

MERC SOL This is absolutely the best homeopathic sore-throat remedy you will find, particularly when your sore throat is accompanied by bad breath, ulcers and/or bleeding gums.

HEPAR SULPH This remedy is ideal for the kind of sore throat that feels as though you have a fish-bone stuck in your throat.

PHYTOLACCA If your sore throat is particularly painful as you swallow and if it is accompanied by general aching in your limbs and your back, this remedy will prove particularly effective.

BELLADONNA This remedy is great if you have a dry, red sore throat that is accompanied by a fever.

KALI MUR Kali mur is excellent for the form of ulcerated sore throat that results from gastric disturbances and when the glands around your throat are swollen.

NUTRITIONAL ADVICE

Always follow the general healthy-eating guidelines on pages 34–35 when trying to beat any infection, including a sore throat. Certain foods are especially good to eat when you have a sore throat as they have particular immune-boosting or soothing properties (see below). Try to increase in or add them to your diet as soon as your symptoms appear. In addition, avoid immune-depleting foods and drinks, such as junk food, alcohol, carbonated drinks and coffee. (Note: If you are a smoker, make this a time to quit. Smoking while you have a sore throat will irritate the mucous membranes in the linings of your lungs and throat making your symptoms much worse.)

FOODS TO EAT

Thyme and cinnamon will help to provide antiseptic properties, while ginger will provide a good anti-inflammatory. Increase your intake of potent immune-boosters, too – garlic, shiitake mushrooms, oranges and other citrus fruits and all fresh fruits and vegetables (especially sweet potatoes, which are particularly high in antioxidants). And eat plenty of soothing Chicken Soup (see recipe, opposite), which not only provides great comfort food, but also helps to fortify your immunity against the infection and soothe the respiratory tract.

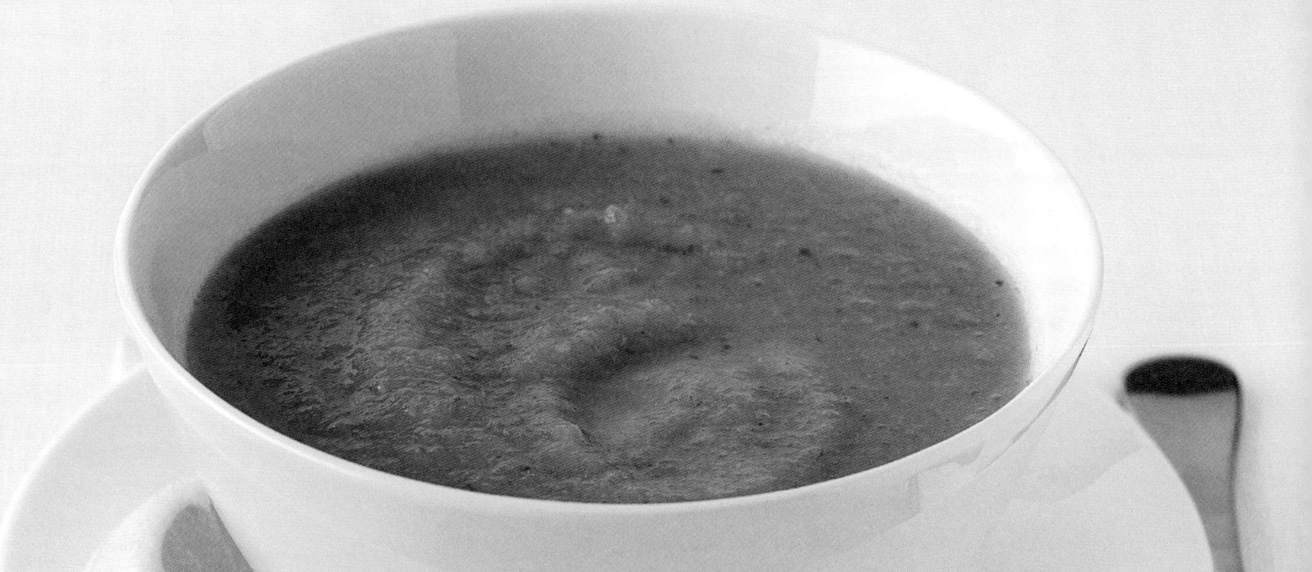

recipe for the throat: **Chicken Soup**

It may seem like an old wives' tale, but scientific research suggests that chicken soup really does help to heal the body as it fights a throat infection. The evidence shows that it works by preventing inflammation in the upper respiratory tract. Here's my very own delicious recipe for chicken soup.

1 x 2–3kg/5–6lb organic whole chicken (without giblets)

2 large onions, chopped

1 large sweet potato, chopped

2 parsnips, chopped

6 large carrots, chopped

3 celery stalks, chopped

1 bunch parsley, chopped

lemon wedges, to serve

Salt and pepper to taste

Put the chicken in a large pot and cover it with cold water. Bring to a boil, then add the onions, sweet potato, parsnips and carrots. Boil for about 1$\frac{1}{2}$ hours, topping up the water if necessary. Skim off the fat from the surface of the water, using a ladle, and add the celery and parsley. Simmer the mixture for a further 45 minutes. Remove the chicken (which you can use for a separate meal), then use a handheld blender to whiz the vegetables and stock into a thick soup. Season with salt and pepper and serve with lemon wedges. Eat as often as you like! (Makes 4–6 servings.)

mouth ulcers

A mouth ulcer is a white or yellow open sore in the mouth. It is usually inflamed and painful, and open to infection from the bacteria naturally found in the mouth.

The Treatment Program

This program tackles the two main causes of mouth ulcers: irritation to the lining of the mouth (such as by abrasive tooth-brushing or sharp teeth) and poor immunity.

RECOMMENDED HERBS

Use the following herbs in a mouthwash or gargle four times a day until the ulcers disappear. Use 10 drops of each tincture in 10ml (2 tsp) water to make the gargle.

CALENDULA (*Calendula officinalis*) Calendula reduces inflammation and assists with tissue repair. It also acts as an antimicrobial, disinfecting the local area.
PROPOLIS (*Resina propoli*) Research shows that flavonoids in propolis give this substance antiseptic, antibiotic, antibacterial, antifungal and antiviral properties.
ST JOHN'S WORT (*Hypericum perforatum*) This wonder herb is rich in anti-inflammatory and antioxidant flavonoids. It is also wound-healing and pain-relieving.
MYRRH (*Commiphora myrrha*) The resin myrrh stimulates the body's production of white blood cells to boost immunity. It is also antimicrobial to beat infection.

SUPPLEMENTARY HERBS

Take 15 drops of each tincture in a little water three times a day to boost your immunity.
• cat's claw (see p.58) • echinacea (see p.58) • goldenseal (see p.58) • olive leaf (see p.60)

ESSENTIAL SUPPLEMENTS

CO-ENZYME Q10 If your mouth ulcers are a result of poor gum health, take a supplement of Co-enzyme Q10 (CoQ10), which can significantly reduce gum disease.
DOSAGE 30mg, daily

right: St John's wort (*Hypericum perforatum*)

ADDITIONAL SUPPLEMENTS

Also take the following immune-boosters until the ulcer has gone.

• vitamin (ester) C (500mg, three times daily; see p.62) • zinc (15g, twice daily; see p.62)

RECOMMENDED HOMEOPATHIC REMEDIES

Use a 6c or 30c potency of each of the following homeopathic remedies up to four times a day until the ulcer has gone.

MERC SOL This is the number-one remedy for mouth ulcers.
ARSEN ALB Arsen alb is great if a hot drink relieves the burning sensation of the ulcer.

NUTRITIONAL ADVICE

Follow the advice on pages 34–35. In addition, avoid eating pineapple and papaya as their enzymatic activity can irritate ulcers; as well as vinegar, pickles and other sour foods (which may irritate the mouth); and acidic foods, such as tomatoes and oranges.

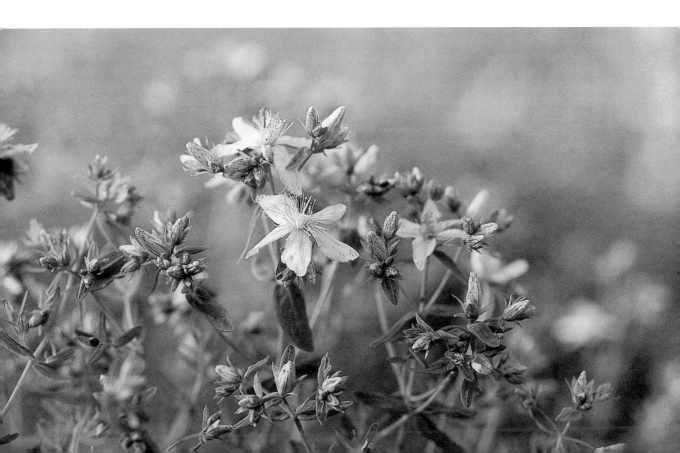

star ingredient: propolis

Used by the ancient Greeks to heal sores and by the ancient Egyptians in embalming, propolis is not strictly a herb, but a resin. Trees such as the poplar, pine, spruce, willow and birch produce this resin, which oozes from the buds and bark. Bees see the propolis, collect it and mix it with nectar and beeswax to use as a glue that both seals the hive against the wind and cold, and (owing to wonderful antiseptic properties) sterilizes it. The product that we collect from the hives is dark green or brown and sticky, with a distinctive medicinal taste. I find it invaluable as a natural remedy because it is a highly effective but gentle wound-healer and a superb anti-aging treatment.

Understanding Propolis

Extensive research has revealed that this resin's most powerful healing properties come from its high concentration of biological, phenolic compounds (natural antiseptics, now frequently used in many conventional medicines). In all, scientists have isolated more than 180 different active constituents in propolis – and we know that there are still more to find.

FOR HEALTH

TO FIGHT ILLNESS Researchers in Poland and Russia have found that propolis directly stimulates the immune system to destroy harmful invading bacteria; while other tests have shown it to be active against viral and fungal infections, too. A great friend to immunity, propolis helps the body to form antibodies, which the immune system uses to identify and disarm pathogens. However, as well as acting as an immuno-stimulant, propolis also contains a high number of phenolic compounds, which themselves help to kill invading bacteria and fungi. In addition, other compounds in propolis, including flavonoids (which occur naturally in many plants or plant-derivatives) may interfere with the movement of bacteria in the body, preventing these pathogens from spreading infection.

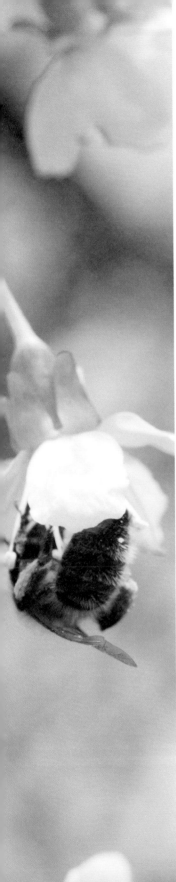

Viruses work by releasing their toxins into our system when enzymatic activity in the body dissolves a protein coat that surrounds the virus cells. The flavonoids in propolis prevent the enzymes from breaking down the protein coat, thereby protecting the body from attack by the virus.

TO CLEANSE WOUNDS Its wide range of anti-pathogenic activity (see above) makes propolis an excellent first-aid cleanser for any open wound on the skin or in the mouth. For small cuts or wounds, combine it as a spray with calendula (see pp.126–127) and St John's wort (see pp.138–139). Use equal measures of each tincture for the mixture. For large areas, dilute the propolis, calendula and St John's wort mixture with cooled, once-boiled water (one part mixture to ten parts water) and wipe the formula over the whole area. You can also use propolis on its own diluted in water (one part propolis to ten parts water) as an antiseptic mouthwash for bleeding gums or mouth ulcers, or after dental surgery.

TO RELIEVE PAIN German researchers have found that, when you apply propolis locally to pain, compounds in its resin possess anesthetic activity.

FOR THE SKIN

TO REDUCE INFLAMMATION Several components in propolis (rather than simply the flavonoids or phenolic compounds) are thought to give the resin a fantastic anti-inflammatory action, by reducing the body's production of the prostaglandins that cause swelling. This makes propolis an excellent choice for topical treatment if you have an inflammatory skin condition, such as eczema or rosacea.

TO REPAIR TISSUE AND HEAL WOUNDS The nutrients and amino acids in propolis contribute to tissue repair. By strengthening blood vessels and promoting the formation of collagen (see p.194), propolis helps skin wounds to heal, whether they are a result of a condition such as eczema or psoriasis, or a cut or graze.

TO REDUCE THE SIGNS OF AGING For all the reasons that propolis works as a good wound-healer, it is also a great anti-aging treatment. In addition, scientists have found that the anti-inflammatory and antioxidant actions of propolis protect the body's cells – including its skin cells – from deterioration, helping to keep the skin younger-looking for longer.

ear infections

Also known as otitis media (infection of the middle ear), ear infections are usually the result of poor immunity. Bacteria or a virus in the Eustachian tube (which connects the middle ear to the back of the nose and throat) cause inflammation and a build-up of a mucousy fluid, leading to pain and fever. Most ear infections are viral, but see your doctor if you have earache, as bacterial infections may need medication.

The Treatment Program

This program aims to fight infection, relieve pain and boost immunity. In addition, it aims to reduce inflammation in the ear and to clear any accumulated mucus.

RECOMMENDED HERBS

For the quickest and most effective results, take the following herbs singly or in combination at the first signs of illness, and in conjunction with homeopathic remedies. Take 15 drops of each tincture diluted in a little water or juice, four times a day.

PLANTAIN (*Plantago major*) Plantain will help to clear mucus from the ear and relieve earache. It also contains the anti-inflammatory flavonoid apigenin.

treating childhood ear infections

The following homeopathic remedies are suitable for children of all ages. Give the herbal tincture only once your child is one year of age or over.

Pulsatilla Give one 200c pillule up to five times a day until the illness has gone.

Sinus and catarrh homeopathic pills These will help to clear mucus. Give one 30c pillule up to five times a day until the infection has gone.

Immune-boosting tincture To fight infection, give 5 drops astragalus **or** elderberry tincture in a little water or juice up to three times a day for a week.

MULLEIN (*Verbascum thapsus*) Like plantain, this pain-relieving antiviral contains apigenin to reduce inflammation. It also soothes irritated mucous membranes.

ELDERBERRY (*Sambucus nigra*) The berries of the elder tree contain compounds that help to reduce inflammation. (The flowers have decongestant properties, which can help if your ear infection is accompanied by a cold or the flu.)

SUPPLEMENTARY HERBS

To boost your immunity against the ear infection, take the following immune-boosting herbs at the first signs of illness and for the duration of the infection:

• astragalus (see p.58) • echinacea (see p.58)

ESSENTIAL SUPPLEMENTS

Increase your intake of the following immune-boosting supplements during the course of the infection. Vitamin C will also support the health of the mucous membranes.

• vitamin (ester) C (500mg, four times daily; see p.62) • zinc (15mg, twice daily; see p.62)

RECOMMENDED HOMEOPATHIC REMEDIES

Use all the following homeopathic remedies from the first signs of illness until the infection has gone. Take a 30c or 200c potency of each, up to five times a day.

MERC SOL If your earache is accompanied by mouth ulcers or bad breath, merc sol is a particularly good remedy.

HEPAR SULPH An excellent remedy if there is pus or discharge from your ear.

ABC (aconite, belladonna, chamomilla) I always keep ABC mixture in the medicine cabinet, because it is excellent for treating ear and other pain, and lowering a fever.

NUTRITIONAL ADVICE

Follow the advice for foods to eat and avoid on page 61. Keep your fluid intake up and boost your vitamin C by drinking plenty of freshly squeezed orange juice, which you should dilute with water. Steer clear of dairy products (except for cottage cheese and plain bio yogurt), which can be mucus-forming.

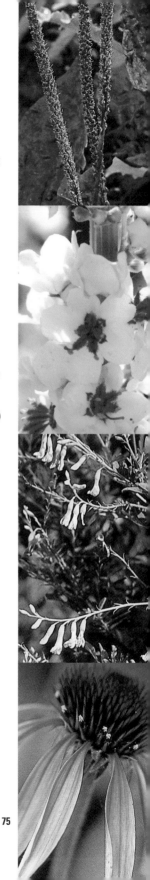

coughs

The lungs are made up of a system of airways called bronchial tubes, which are lined with cells that secrete mucus. The mucus traps any particles that may enter the lungs when we breathe in, and these particles are then swept out of the lungs by tiny hairs, called cilia, that also line the airways. When something irritates the bronchial lining – perhaps because of an infection, a smoky environment, or a condition such as asthma – the lungs produce excess mucus. This in turn causes a spasmodic cough that is designed to expel the extra mucus and anything trapped in it.

The Treatment Program

Coughs are notoriously difficult to treat. However, I have found several herbs and homeopathic remedies to be particularly effective at easing respiration and overcoming the cough – sometimes within only a few days. All the remedies I've given are relevant for coughs no matter what their cause, unless I have specifically said otherwise.

RECOMMENDED HERBS

The following combination of herbs can see a cough disappear within two days if you take them promptly at the first signs of infection. Take 15 drops of each tincture in a little water or juice, three times a day until the cough has gone.

ELECAMPANE (*Inula helenium*) This herb activates the tissue of the upper respiratory tract to help you to bring up excess mucus, creating a stimulating but gentle expectorant. Elecampane also reduces bronchial spasms, meaning that it eases coughing, and also acts as an antibacterial agent if the cough is infection-related.

COLTSFOOT (*Tussilago farfara*) Coltsfoot is an effective antitussive because it contains mucilage, bitter glycosides, and tannins, which work together to soothe the irritated mucous membranes and reduce inflammation in the airways of the lungs.

LUNGWORT (*Pulmonaria officinalis*) Soothing and antispasmodic, lungwort can be particularly effective at reducing a nighttime cough, so relieving disturbed sleep.

right: lungwort (*Pulmonaria officinalis*)

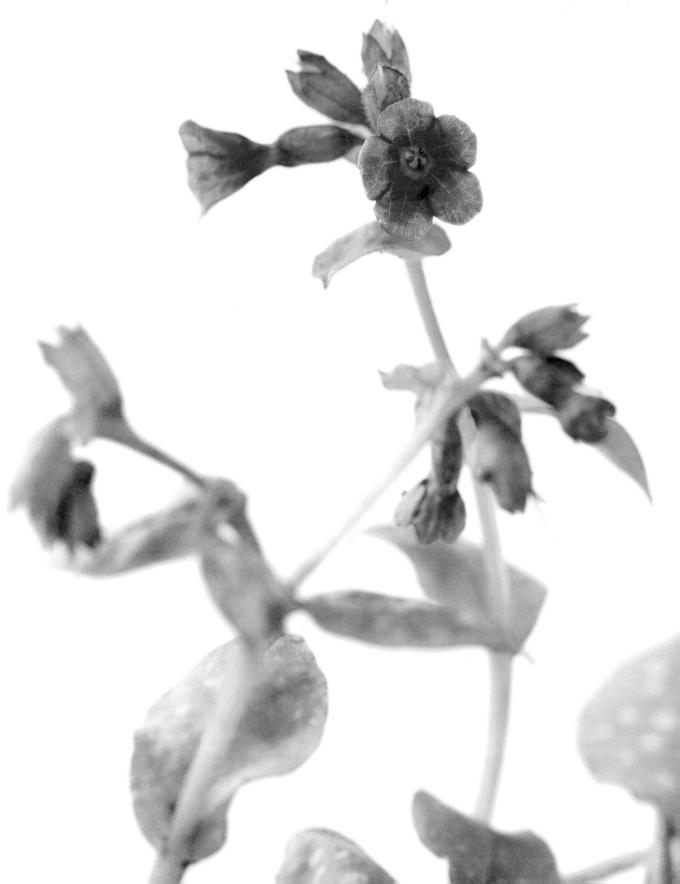

LICORICE (*Glycyrrhiza glabra*) This soothing expectorant contains glycyrrhizinic acid, which helps to reduce inflammation in the mucous membranes that line the airways.
MULLEIN (*Verbascum thapsus*) Mullein soothes the throat and the bronchial passages. Classed as a relaxing reflex expectorant, this herb helps to ease congestion by reducing the viscosity of mucous secretions (phlegm), making them easier to expel.

ESSENTIAL SUPPLEMENTS

As the lungs are an important part of our immune system, it is crucial to get them into prime health quickly. Increase the dosage of these immune-boosting supplements as follows for the duration of your cough, then return to your normal dosage.
• vitamin (ester) C (500mg, four times daily; see p.62) • zinc (15mg, twice daily; see p.62)

RECOMMENDED HOMEOPATHIC REMEDIES

When a homeopath treats a cough, he or she will assess your symptoms according to two categories: dry cough and wet cough. A dry cough is the more common and is "unproductive" – that is, it doesn't bring up any phlegm or mucus. A wet cough tends to be the "productive", phlegmy kind. Because the nature of a cough can change so quickly, finding the single, correct remedy can be difficult. Nevertheles, I have found the three combinations opposite to be very useful for treating each type of cough. Take these, alongside my recommended herbs and supplements, in 30c potency up to five times a day for three or four days.

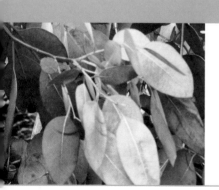

eucalyptus and thyme inhalation

A steam inhalation using eucalyptus and thyme essential oils helps to relieve congestion in the upper respiratory tract by loosening mucus and opening the airways. Both oils also have antibacterial qualities. Add two drops of each oil to a bowl of near-boiling water. Remove your spectacles if you wear them, then lean over the bowl. Cover your head and the bowl with a towel and inhale the steam.

treating childhood coughs

The following variation of the adult treatment program works wonders with my own children – often reducing a cough that would probably have lasted three weeks to one that lasts just two days. This program is suitable for children aged two and over. (Children aged ten and over can be treated as adults.)

Sinus and catarrh homeopathic pills Widely available at natural health stores, these will help to reduce the yellow or green mucus in the chest and nose. Give one 30c pill four times a day until the cough has gone.

Cough and mucus tincture Combine five drops of each of the herbal tinctures in the adult program and give your child the mixture in a little water or apple juice, four times a day for one week.

DRY COUGH MIXTURE (bryonia, spongia, drosera, sticta pulmonaria) This mixture combines three remedies widely valued for their ability to treat dry coughs.

WET COUGH MIXTURE (hepar sulph and ant tart) This mixture combines remedies that are commonly used to treat all kinds of wet cough.

SINUS AND CATARRH MIXTURE (pulsatilla, hepar sulph, merc sol, thuja, hydrastis, kali bich) This is particularly effective if you have a green or yellow phlegmy discharge.

NUTRITIONAL ADVICE

During a cough your diet should boost your immunity and clear mucus from and reduce inflammation in the respiratory system. Other than the usual junk and processed foods, the only foods you really need to avoid are dairy foods (except plain bio yogurt and cottage cheese), which can be mucus-forming.

FOODS TO EAT

Eat plenty of oranges, garlic, shellfish (especially zinc-rich oysters), lemons, onions, broccoli, carrots, nuts and seeds. Drink a cup of green tea a day. Ginger will help to reduce inflammation, while lemon and sweet potato will help to clear mucus.

bloating (gas)

Bloating, accompanied by abdominal swelling is usually the result of excess gas in the large intestine, or colon. In general, 85 percent of gas in your gut is air you have swallowed while eating. The remaining 15 percent is a result of bad bacteria in the intestines or the release of gas from partially digested food that has begun to ferment in the gut.

The Treatment Program

The herbal and homeopathic treatments below will help to relieve the bloating itself, rather than any of its underlying causes – so be sure to change your diet, too!

RECOMMENDED HERBS

Take these herbs singly or in combination at a dosage of 15 drops of each tincture in a little water or juice, three times a day until the bloating and any spasm has gone (unless otherwise directed).

ANISE (*Pimpinella anisum*), NUTMEG (*Myristica fragrans*), CARDAMOM (*Elettaria cardamomum*), CINNAMON (*Cinnamomum zeylanicum*) All these herbs help to break down gas, aid digestion and reduce bloating. If you prefer, you could take this mixture in powder form. Take ¼ tsp, dissolved in a little water, once a day after big meals.
FENNEL (*Foeniculum vulgare*) This herb contains the substance anethole, which helps to ease muscle spasms and cramping and so reduces the build-up of gas in the gut.
PEPPERMINT (*Mentha piperita*) Peppermint helps to relax the muscles in the gut so they release trapped air. (Avoid peppermint if you suffer from constipation.)
GINGER (*Zingiber officinalis*) A digestive cure-all, ginger can reduce muscle spasm.

ESSENTIAL SUPPLEMENTS

Take this combination of supplements specifically when you suffer a bout of bloating. Stop taking them when your gut has returned to normal.

DETOX CAPSULES Many people find that toxicity and bloating often go hand in hand. A detox will greatly help the gut and quickly relieve bloating. (See pp.41–55 for information on how to detox.)

DOSAGE Three capsules every morning and evening.

PROBIOTICS "Good" bacteria can help to reduce the risk of food fermenting in the gut.

DOSAGE Two billion, twice daily.

DIGESTIVE ENZYMES, AND CALCIUM AND MAGNESIUM COMPLEX These two supplements relieve stress on the digestive tract and improve the symptoms of gas.

DOSAGE Follow the dosage instructions on the label for the digestive enzymes and take 1,000mg daily of the calcium and magnesium complex.

RECOMMENDED HOMEOPATHIC REMEDIES

Take these homeopathic remedies at a potency of 30c or 200c, three times a day.

CARBO VEG, NUX VOM, LYCOPODIUM These remedies can help to relieve the symptoms of bloating. See Irritable Bowel Syndrome (pp.102–105).

ARGENT NIT AND GELSEMIUM These remedies are especially helpful if your bloating is accompanied by anxiety and diarrhea.

NUTRITIONAL ADVICE

Remember to chew your food well, as this gets digestion started, and drink water away from mealtimes so as not to dilute your digestive juices.

FOODS TO EAT

Gas-reducing foods include unrefined carbohydrates, such as brown rice and all fruits and vegetables (except those below). Eat foods that contain "good" bacteria, such as plain bio yogurt; and foods, such as papaya, that are rich in digestive enzymes.

FOODS TO AVOID

Avoid cabbage, Brussels sprouts, turnip, and rape (canola) and mustard seed, which tend to be gas-forming. Avoid mucus-forming dairy (except yogurt and cottage cheese).

constipation

Around fifty percent of the people who come to see us at The Organic Pharmacy come about constipation. The condition occurs when the stool becomes soft and lacks bulk and the muscular contractions of the bowel cannot move it along the colon. Conversely, the stool may be healthy, but you may suffer constipation because the bowel is sluggish and doesn't contract well enough to advance the stool along its path. Your body then reabsorbs the water in the stool, making it too hard to pass. Stress, a low-fibre diet, dehydration and inadequate exercise are the main causes of constipation; while pregnancy, toxicity, bowel disease (such as Irritable Bowel Syndrome), iron and calcium supplements, codeine-based drugs (including some painkillers) and drugs containing aluminium are all also common triggers.

The Treatment Program

Regular bowel movements remove toxins from the body. When food and waste are trapped in the colon, the body reabsorbs toxins. This may result in chronic symptoms, such as bloating, cramps, body odour, bad breath and hemorrhoids. Making basic changes to your diet, including eating more fibre-rich foods (such as linseed/flax) that bulk out the stool, often relieves symptoms. In stubborn cases, when even a high-fibre diet fails to bring relief, herbs, supplements and homeopathy can provide the answer.

RECOMMENDED HERBS

TRIPHALA A balanced blend of three Indian fruits – harada, amla and behada – triphala not only has antioxidant activity, but also acts as a mild, natural laxative.
DOSAGE 15 drops tincture in a little water or juice, three times a day.

RECOMMENDED SUPPLEMENTS

Take the following supplements during a bout of constipation (but don't take them all the time as a preventative). Together, they will help to move the stool through the colon and also minimize the risk of toxins being reabsorbed into the circulation.

right: linseed/flax (*Linum usitatissimum*)

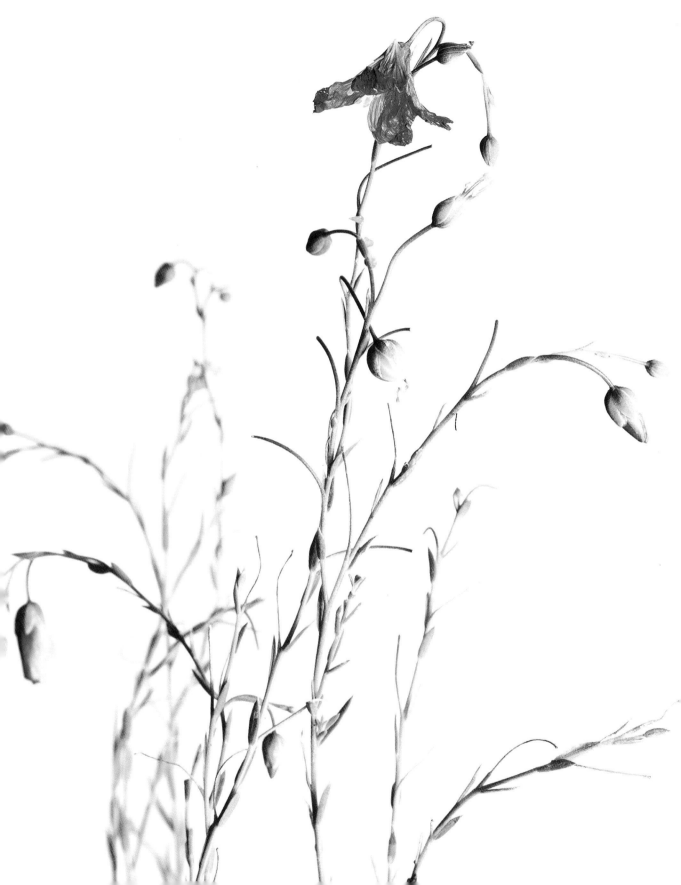

take certain herbs with caution

The herbs cascara, senna and aloe latex are commonly used to treat constipation, but all three contain anthranoid laxatives, which need healthy bowel flora to make them work – and healthy flora are usually lacking in a person with constipation. They draw water into the gut by opening the channels for sodium and chlorine ions (water will always follow). This can cause runny stools and dehydration. These herbs may also trigger a physiological reaction that causes the gut walls to contract, resulting in cramps and diarrhea. Overall, cascara, senna and aloe latex have a strong laxative effect, which in the long term can cause the muscles of the large intestine to become lazy, worsening constipation. Avoid them unless your constipation is severe – in which case take them for only one or two days.

DETOX CAPSULES These contain psyllium, linseed (flax seed) and apple pectin, which clean the gut, providing effective treatment for constipation. The capsules also contain clay, which draws out toxins from the gut. This prevents the gut wall absorbing toxins back into the body to keep the whole system healthy during a bout of constipation.
DOSAGE Two capsules, every morning (and make sure you drink at least eight glasses of water throughout the day).
PROBIOTICS Bowel flora are crucial for helping to keep the gut healthy. In the case of constipation, they help to keep toxic bacteria in check.
DOSAGE Eight billion, daily.
DIGESTIVE ENZYMES Taking a digestive enzyme supplement during a bout of constipation will ensure that all the good nutrients from your food are absorbed into your system, while the toxins stay out.
DOSAGE One capsule ten minutes before lunch and another ten minutes before dinner.

RECOMMENDED HOMEOPATHIC REMEDIES
Take each of the following homeopathic remedies in a 6c potency, three times a day for two days. If they have not worked during this time, and you are still experiencing

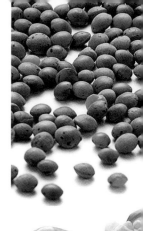

constipation, please seek advice from a registered homeopath, who will be able to give you a formula tailored to your own symptoms and constitution.

ALUMINA This is the number-one homeopathic remedy for constipation as it helps to boost a sluggish bowel, thus moving the stool through the colon.

BRYONIA This remedy is perfect if you have very small, dry stools, and also suffer from dryness in other parts of your body, too – such as dry skin or a dry cough.

SEPIA This remedy will help to relieve the sensation of "bearing down" in the bowel and is particularly good if your constipation is hormone-related.

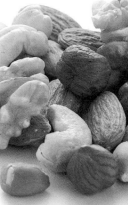

NUTRITIONAL ADVICE

Fibre is the key to overcoming constipation. There are two types – soluble and insoluble fibre – and a healthy stool needs a balance of both. Soluble fibre absorbs water to soften the stool; insoluble fibre does not hold water, but gives the stool bulk, so that it can move quickly through the system.

FOODS TO EAT

Fruits and legumes, as well as psyllium (see p.46), are good sources of soluble fibre, while whole grains and bran are good sources of insoluble fibre. Apples, pears, plums, all vegetables, wholemeal breads and cereals, brown rice, nuts and seeds, and bilberries all give you the kinds of fibre you need for a healthy stool. Make sure you eat plenty of water-rich foods – such as fruit, vegetables, salads and so on – and drink at least eight glasses of water a day, between meals (so as not to dilute your digestive juices). To stimulate the movement of the wall of the large intestine, try eating a daily dose of prunes; and keep up the low-fat plain bio yogurt for all its good bacteria. Pears, figs and rhubarb will all help to soften the stool.

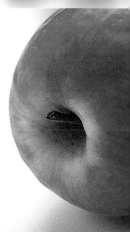

FOODS TO AVOID

Highly refined foods lack the fibre and nutrients needed for good bowel health. So, avoid all "white" products – from bread and pasta to rice. A high-protein, low-carb diet may also lead to constipation.

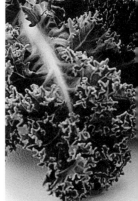

food poisoning

Figures in the UK suggest that the country has almost 80,000 cases of food poisoning every year, while in the US the estimate is around 76 million. The symptoms of food poisoning (diarrhea and vomiting in particular) are signs that the body is trying to expel the pathogens from the system quickly – which is why it's important not to take medication to stop diarrhea.

The Treatment Program

Bacteria (such as *salmonella* or *Staphylococcus aureus*), viruses and parasites in food are the most common causes of food poisoning. However, in rare cases toxins that occur naturally in foods, such as those in uncooked kidney beans, sprouted or green potatoes, and shellfish, as well as low stomach acid (which means the body cannot clean pathogens from food properly), can also cause illness. The following treatment

naturally occurring food toxins

There are some foods that contain "natural" toxins, and when you eat these foods you may experience some of the symptoms of food poisoning. Below I've set out the most common culprits, with some advice on how to minimize or eliminate their effects.

Potatoes The humble potato contains a glycoalkaloid (see p.121) called solanine, which your body converts to the poison solanidine. This poison can, in sensitive people, cause severe stomach cramps. Avoid eating potatoes that have turned green or have sprouted, which cause potatoes to have a particularly high solanine content.

Kidney beans These beans contain toxins called lectins, which can cause vomiting, stomach cramps and diarrhea. In order to remove the lectins, soak the beans in water for four or five hours and then boil them until tender before eating.

Shellfish All shellfish are filter-feeders, which means they ingest toxins in the water. Buy shellfish from a reputable fishmonger and always cook them thoroughly.

program aims to assist the body in its vital work killing and eliminating the pathogens and their toxins. The program doesn't try to stop any diarrhea or vomiting altogether, which would just hamper the body's natural defences.

RECOMMENDED HERBS

Taking anything (including herbs) can be extremely difficult when you have food poisoning. If you can keep anything down, the following herbs can be very helpful.

FOR INFECTION

Take 15 drops each of these tinctures in a little water four times a day during infection.

PAU D'ARCO (*Tabebuia avellanedae*) This herb is a highly effective antimicrobial and antiparasitic, assisting the body in its fight against invading pathogens.
GOLDENSEAL (*Hydrastis canadensis*) Goldenseal has an antibiotic-like action against food-poisoning pathogens such as *E. coli*, *shigelia*, *salmonella* and *giardia*.

FOR THE SYSTEM

Take 15 drops of each of the following herbal tinctures, three times a day for a week once the diarrhea and vomiting have stopped.
GINGER (*Zingiber officinalis*) Ginger contains shogaols and gingerols, which are thought to normalize the contractions of the digestive tract, helping to stop cramps.
MILK THISTLE (*Sylibum marianum*) As toxins are often to blame in bouts of food poisoning, this super-detox herb is perfect for boosting the efficiency of the liver – one of our main organs of detoxification – by helping with its cell regeneration.
OLIVE LEAF (*Olea europaea*) Olive leaf contains a bitter phytochemical compound called oleuropein, which attacks bacteria and fungi and dissolves their outer membrane, thereby preventing them replicating.

ESSENTIAL SUPPLEMENTS

Take the first three of these supplements as soon as you are able to keep anything down. Then, take the probiotics as soon as you show signs of recovery.

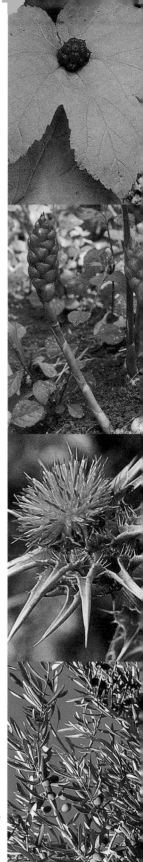

APPLE CIDER VINEGAR This supplement helps to normalize the acidity in the stomach and to kill harmful bacteria. It also aids digestion and soothes stomach spasms.

DOSAGE Once a day, take 1 tbsp apple cider vinegar in a small glass of water sweetened with 1 tsp honey, until sickness or diarrhea has gone.

GRAPEFRUIT SEED EXTRACT This potent antimicrobial is active against bacteria, viruses and yeasts, including some of the main culprits of food poisoning, such as *salmonella*, *giardia*, *lysteria* and *Helicobacter pylori*.

DOSAGE Two capsules as soon as possible once the poisoning has started, then take at least three more doses over the course of your illness.

DETOX CAPSULES Pectin and clay (contained in detox capsules) are very effective at mopping up toxins and eliminating them from the system quickly. Chlorella is excellent at helping to get rid of heavy metals, in particular mercury, from the body.

DOSAGE Three capsules, three times a day for three days.

PROBIOTICS Any kind of diarrhea or infection in the gut will disturb the balance of the bowel flora. This gives the bad bacteria an opportunity to take over and colonize in place of the good bacteria. Probiotics are friendly bacteria that help to recolonize your gut, rather than letting the bad flora take over.

DOSAGE Eight billion a day, for three days.

travelbug first aid

There's nothing worse than a bad tummy while you are travelling. If you're visiting a zone where food poisoning is common, take the following herbal remedy beginning two days before you go and every day for the duration of your trip: combine equal parts of the tinctures of goldenseal, milk thistle and olive leaf, and dilute 15 drops of the mixture in a glass of clean, pure water. Also, make sure you take your daily dosage of two billion probiotics, as well as two capsules of grapefruit seed extract also every day. These will help to kill pathogens and boost immunity so that even if you do get food poisoning, the effects will not be as severe. It is useful to take your homeopathic food-poisoning combination (see p.90) just in case.

right: olive (*Olea europaea*)

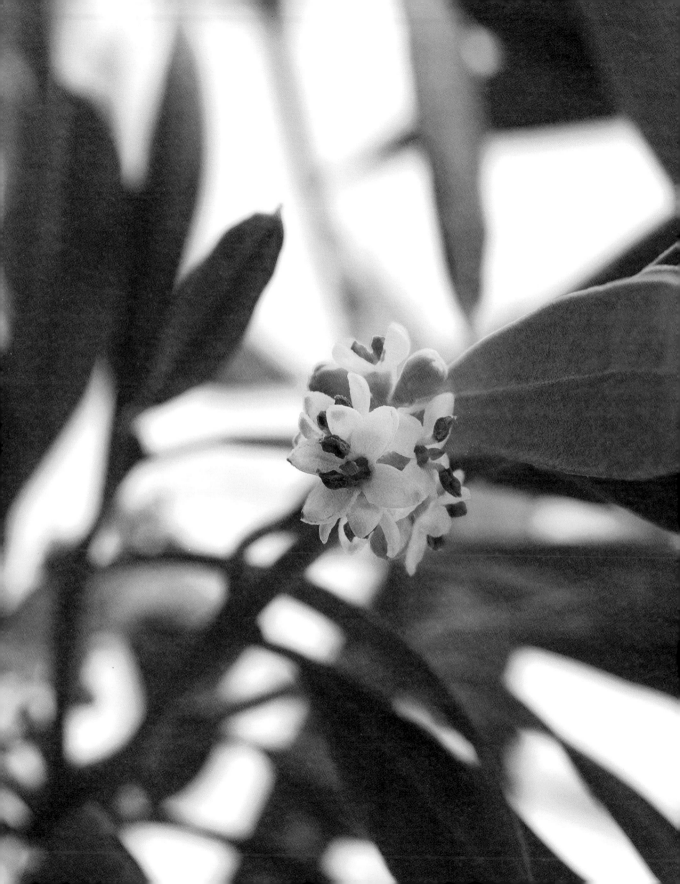

RECOMMENDED HOMEOPATHIC REMEDIES

Homeopathic remedies not only help the body to overcome illness quickly, but they also stay down easily – and even help with vomiting. You can take the remedies singly or as a combination. Take a 6c or 30c potency of each every 15 minutes from the first signs of symptoms, and gradually tailor off the frequency as your symptoms improve.

ARSEN ALB This number-one food-poisoning remedy helps to ease the typical symptoms of food poisoning, including nausea, vomiting and diarrhea.

MAG PHOS This is the best remedy for the relief of cramping.

CHINA (CHINCHONA) China helps to relieve cramps and ease vomiting.

CARBO VEG If your vomiting and diarrhea are accompanied by gas and bloating, this homeopathic remedy will help to ease the extra symptoms.

NUX VOM This remedy will ease vomiting and cramps without suppressing the body's natural desire to expel the toxins.

NUTRITIONAL ADVICE

Vomiting and diarrhea result in huge amounts of water loss, so make sure you keep drinking filtered water – even if it is a sip at a time. To replace minerals, in particular salts and bicarbonate, take an electrolyte supplement (available at most pharmacies).

FOODS TO EAT

Once any vomiting subsides and the digestive tract calms down, for the first few days eat only plain boiled rice, light vegetable or tiny pasta soups, dry crackers or dry toast, and low-fat plain bio yogurt (to boost your beneficial bacteria). Most importantly, don't eat more than you feel you can – little and often is best. Reintroduce foods slowly once your digestive system has had 48 to 72 hours to recover.

FOODS TO AVOID

At least until you are completely recovered, avoid fried, heavy or creamy foods, raw vegetables (which your body will find difficult to digest), meat, and alcohol (which will dehydrate you).

diarrhea

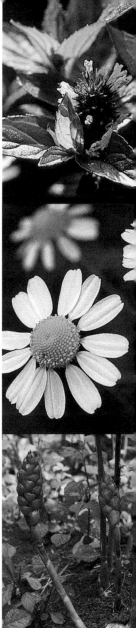

Diarrhea need not always be caused by infection – it may be a symptom of non-infectious diseases such as Irritable Bowel Syndrome (IBS) or Crohn's disease, as well as of conditions such as food intolerance or nervousness.

The Treatment Program

The following are the ideal remedies for treating non-infection-related diarrhea. Also take the supplements given for IBS (see p.104), but avoid grapefruit seed extract.

RECOMMENDED HERBS

Take 15 drops of the following herbal tinctures in a little water, three times a day during chronic diarrhea, or as necessary for diarrhea caused by anxiety.

PEPPERMINT (*Mentha piperita*) Antispasmodic peppermint is well known for its ability to calm the stomach and relieve diarrhea. It also helps to reduce stomach gas.
GERMAN CHAMOMILE (*Matricaria recutita*) This herb contains various compounds that help to calm the gut, reducing inflammation and spasms, and relieving diarrhea.
GINGER (*Zingiber officinalis*) Ginger is anti-spasmodic and calming for the stomach.

RECOMMENDED HOMEOPATHIC REMEDIES

Take each of the following remedies in a potency of 6c or 30c as often as you need to.

ALOE, ARSEN ALB, IRIS, PODOPHYLLUM This combination has proven to be very useful in the treatment of the symptoms of diarrhea.
ARGENT NIT, LYCOPODIUM, GELSEMIUM These remedies are particularly effective when your symptoms are related to anxiety, including performance-related diarrhea.

NUTRITIONAL ADVICE

Follow the nutritional advice given for Irritable Bowel Syndrome (see p.105).

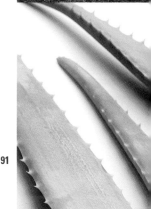

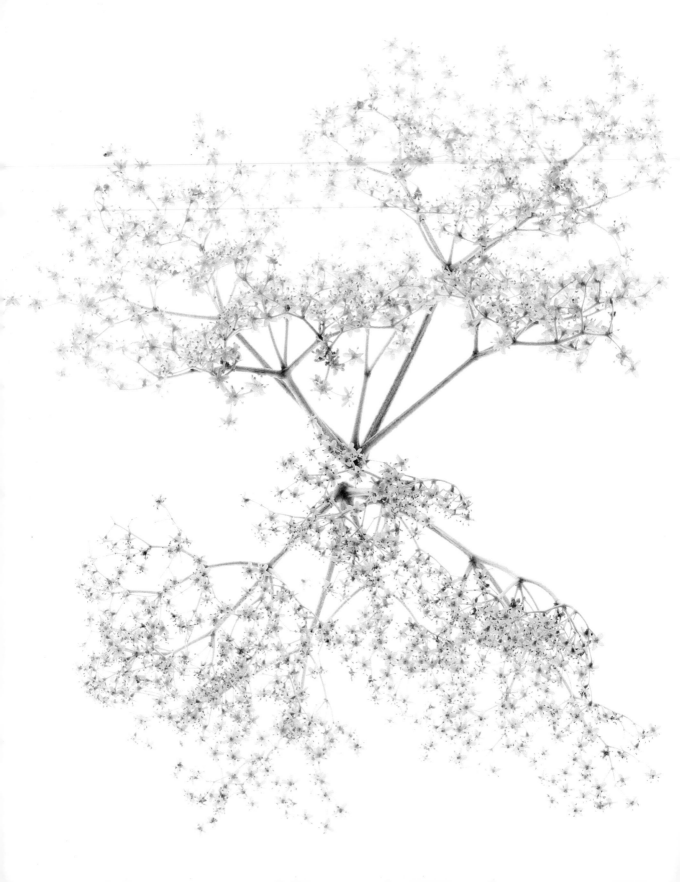

healing chronic complaints

A chronic illness is a long-term condition that lasts three months or more and may recur. Candida, insomnia, stress, hay fever and Irritable Bowel Syndrome (IBS) are all examples of chronic conditions.

Many chronic illnesses are signs of lowered immunity. In these cases, any treatment plan must first look at boosting immunity so that your body can restore its natural equilibrium and bring you to a state of health. Other chronic illnesses are auto-immune conditions. These are the conditions that we commonly call allergies, and that include hay fever. For these, you should avoid immune-boosting remedies and instead look to calm the immune system.

All of the conditions in this chapter feature a program based on my three-pronged approach. However, although each one has a list of homeopathic remedies, it is especially important when treating a chronic condition to have a private consultation with a registered homeopath, who will look at your constitution and symptoms and then prescribe treatments that are tailored to you. In order to give every treatment program the best chance of success, I also recommend that, with the blessing of your doctor or other healthcare professional, you follow the ten-day detox (see pp.50–53) every three months to ensure that your body is primed to work at its optimum levels.

left: elderflower (*Sambucus nigra*)

candida (yeast infections)

Candida albicans **is a fungus (or yeast) that is naturally present in your body. Your immune system usually keeps it in check through the work of the good bacteria in your gut. When something kills off the good bacteria or encourages the growth of the bad, the candida fungus multiplies. In time, this can lead to conditions such as candidiasis, thrush, athlete's foot and fungal nail.**

The Treatment Program

At The Organic Pharmacy, at least one in every three people we see is infected with candida, and almost every case of food intolerance or allergy has candidiasis as the

how the flora become imbalanced

So what can trigger an imbalance between the good and the bad flora in the body, leading to conditions such as candidiasis?

Antibiotics These kill off all bacteria – including the friendly bacteria – in your gut.

Toxicity in the gut Toxicity causes a sluggish digestive system, which means that food remains in the gut for too long and begins to ferment, providing a hospitable breeding ground for the bad flora at the expense of the good.

Sugar (including alchohol) and refined carbohydrates All forms of sugar and refined carbs, such as white pasta, bread and rice, give candida plenty of food to thrive on, helping the fungi to colonize the gut.

Yeast foods It stands to reason that if you eat fungal foods (including foods that have invisible fungi in them, such as nuts and dried fruit), you will add to the level of bad flora in your body.

Hormonal imbalance Synthetic estrogens, such as those in the contraceptive pill and even their residues in tapwater, can promote the growth of bad flora in the gut.

main underlying cause. To combat the problem, you need to balance your gut by making its environment less friendly to candida. I recommend taking probiotic supplements and following a low-sugar, low-yeast diet. You can also directly kill the fungus with antifungal herbs and supplements.

RECOMMENDED HERBS

Combine 15 drops of the tinctures of each of the following herbs in a small amount of water or juice and take this remedy three times a day.

PAU D'ARCO (*Tabebuia avellanedae*) This antimicrobial and immunity-boosting herb contains compounds called napthaquinones – potent antifungals.

GOLDENSEAL (*Hydrastis canadensis*) Goldenseal contains the alkaloid berberine, which hinders the growth of candida. Never take goldenseal for more than two weeks at a time with a two-week break, unless supervised by a registered practitioner.

OLIVE LEAF (*Olea europaea*) Oleuropein, a bitter phytochemical in olive leaf, attacks fungi and prevents replication. Olive leaf is also an effective immunity-booster.

ECHINACEA (*Echinacea purpurea*) The number-one immunity herb, echinacea increases the body's production of white blood cells, which attack invading organisms, including bacteria, viruses and fungi.

ESSENTIAL SUPPLEMENTS

PROBIOTICS Good bacteria, such as acidophilus, help to prevent the overgrowth of the candida fungus in the gut, as well as generally boosting the immune system.
DOSAGE Eight billion, daily.

GRAPEFRUIT SEED EXTRACT This supplement attacks the cell membranes of the candida fungus so the cell's contents escape, thereby inactivating the fungus.
DOSAGE One capsule, three times a day.

DETOX CAPSULES As it dies off, the candida fungus produces toxins that may cause headaches, nausea and fatigue. Detox capsules absorb and eliminate these toxins.
DOSAGE Three capsules thirty minutes before breakfast and another three before bedtime, every day until the infection has gone.

ESSENTIAL FATTY ACIDS AND B-COMPLEX VITAMINS This combined supplement provides nutrients that are essential for your body if it is to resist the yeast infection. *DOSAGE* Three capsules every day with breakfast until symptoms subside.

RECOMMENDED HOMEOPATHIC REMEDIES

Candida is not a straightforward condition to treat with homeopathy, but there are two remedies I have found to be really useful for relieving the symptoms of both genital thrush and oral thrush. They are also suitable for babies and pregnant women.

treating topical conditions

There is a strong likelihood that if you have candida internally, you will also have a related skin condition, such as athlete's foot, fungal nail, thrush, oral thrush, ringworm or dandruff. Once you begin internal treatment, you should expect your topical symptoms to get worse, because the body pushes the fungus out of the body via the mouth, skin and vagina. This is normal and nothing to be concerned about, but there are treatments you can take to ease the process. Plants and trees protect themselves from damaging mould by producing potent antifungal extracts that we can collect and use topically. The most effective are the essential oils of tea tree, manuka and neem, and the tinctures of calendula and propolis. I confess that many of these extracts really do not smell good – in particular neem and manuka oils – but they do work. The following are the treatments I recommend.

For the skin and vagina (externally) Use a cream with manuka, neem and tea tree oil.

For the mouth Dilute 10 drops of each of calendula and propolis tinctures in a little water and use as a mouthwash at least three times a day, or as often as you can. Or, make a mouthwash with a citricidal liquid (such as grapefruit seed extract), diluted according to the packet instructions, but be warned that it has a very bitter taste.

For nail infections Rub the affected area with a little neem oil every day. This is a highly effective remedy but you have to be patient – it can take at least four months to eradicate nail fungus.

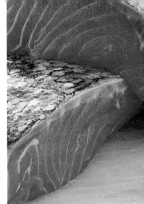

BORAX AND KREOSOTUM These are both effective remedies for vaginal itching with discharge, and they are also useful for combatting oral thrush. Use them in conjunction with the recommended nutritional program below.

POTENCY 6c *DOSAGE* Four times a day.

NUTRITIONAL ADVICE

Candida is a complex fungal infection to treat, so rather than recommending individual foods for you to increase in your diet, I prefer to recommend food groups that will help to balance the flora in your gut, keep toxicity at bay, and make your body inhospitable to the fungus. In addition, there are several foods you should avoid, because they will provide a fungal breeding ground. Follow this eating plan for between three and four months. You may experience detox symptoms (such as headaches or pimples) to begin with, but don't be alarmed – this is normal and shows the program is working.

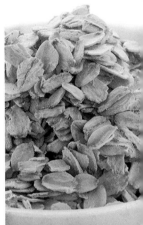

FOODS TO EAT

As well as eating lots of fresh, organic vegetables and proteins (eggs, meat and fish), make your diet as yeast-free as possible. Eat good-quality, yeast-free rye or wholegrain bread that has been freshly baked that day and not stored in a plastic bag. Eat wholegrain rye, oats and quinoa, which are yeast-free. And eat plenty of low-fat plain bio yogurt, which will boost your "good" gut flora.

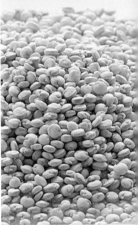

FOODS TO AVOID

Avoid sugar in all its guises – including fruit juices and refined carbohydrates, such as white pasta, white bread and white rice. Dried fruits are out, too, because these are high in sugar and often mouldy (even if you can't see the mould). Coffee, tea and plastic-packed sliced bread are likely to grow mould (again, even when you can't see it), so steer clear of these; and avoid any yeast foods – for example, fermented foods (such as soy, vinegar and malt) and bread. Avoid fungal foods, such as mushrooms, although make shiitake mushrooms an exception because they are great for your immunity. Finally, put away the mouldy cheeses – blue cheese, soft cheese with a rind (such as Brie), and hard cheese that has gone mouldy.

hay fever

Your immune system protects you from harmful pathogens such as bacteria and viruses to keep you healthy. However, in some people, the immune system is oversensitive and responds to substances that are harmless. Hay fever (properly called seasonal allergic rhinitis) is the immune system's over-reaction to pollen and plant spores in the air. These allergens trigger the body's production of antibodies, which then prompts the release of the messenger chemical histamine. This response causes the itchy, watery, red eyes, and the runny nose, sneezing, fatigue, headache and coughing that are symptomatic of hay fever.

The Treatment Program

Balancing out the immune response, so that your immune system does not over-react to plant material, is the primary way to relieve long-term suffering from hay fever. However, there are also many herbs and other treatments that will help you to cope with the symptoms of the condition. Usually, it's specific pollens that trigger a reaction in each individual. Try to pinpoint when you experience the first signs of your hay fever. Then, begin the treatment program two to three months beforehand.

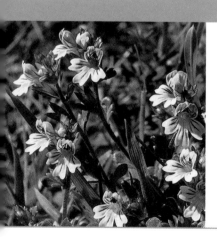

soothing your eyes

Homeopathic eye drops can prove very useful in easing the stinging, itching eye symptoms of hay fever. There are several excellent ready-made drops available from good natural pharmacies. (The same is true for nasal sprays, to ease congestion.) Alternatively, dilute 1 drop euphrasia tincture in an eye bath filled with cooled, boiled water and rinse one eye. Then, using fresh mixture, repeat the process on the other eye (you don't have to have a sterile eye bath for the other eye, as you aren't treating an infection).

RECOMMENDED HERBS

Many anti-inflammatory herbs are effective anti-histamines, and some can help break up mucus and expel it. Take 15 drops of each of the following tinctures in a little water or juice, three times a day (unless otherwise stated) from spring to the end of summer.

GERMAN CHAMOMILE (*Matricaria recutita*) A variety of active compounds in German chamomile work in synergy to reduce inflammation in the eyes, nose and throat, strengthen the mucous membranes, and prevent the release of histamine.

ELDERFLOWER (*Sambucus nigra*) These flowers are rich in flavonoids and triterpenes, which give them anti-inflammatory and anti-catarrhal properties.

NETTLE (*Urtica dioica*) Nettle leaves contain formic acid and histamine (which acts homeopathically), helping to alleviate itching eyes, sneezing and mucus production.

EYEBRIGHT (*Euphrasia officinalis*) A strong anti-inflammatory for the eyes, nose and other mucous membranes, eyebright helps to reduce swelling, and has anti-catarrhal and astringent properties, which help to soothe sore eyes and a tender nose.

HOW TO USE Fill an eye bath with cooled, boiled water and put in 1 drop eyebright tincture. Rinse one eye thoroughly; then repeat the process in the other eye.

ESSENTIAL SUPPLEMENTS

QUERCETIN The number-one supplement for hay-fever sufferers, quercetin acts by inhibiting the production and release of histamine.

DOSAGE 400–500mg, twice daily.

BROMELAIN AND VITAMIN (ESTER) C Bromelain is an enzyme that occurs naturally in vegetables. Both bromelain and vitamin C are highly effective anti-inflammatories.

DOSAGE 500–1,000mg, twice daily.

ESSENTIAL FATTY ACIDS These will promote tissue-repair in the cells of the nose and throat, and help to reduce inflammation.

DOSAGE 100mg, twice daily.

In addition, be sure to take your daily antioxidant supplement (see p.21). This will protect your cells from damage caused by inflammation and reduce inflammation itself.

RECOMMENDED HOMEOPATHIC REMEDIES

I can't stress enough how important it is to see a homeopath two months or so in advance of the onset of your symptoms. The homeopath will be able to work at a deep, constitutional level that is unique to you to help prevent or reduce your symptoms before they begin to appear. Following the homeopath's advice, year after year, will hopefully see all your symptoms completely gone within a few years. Even without an individual consultation, there are many remedies that will help to control and reduce hay-fever symptoms. Take the following in a 6c or 30c potency up to six times a day until your personal hay-fever season is over.

HAY FEVER COMPLEX (euphrasia, sabadilla, allium cepa, nat mur, histamine, arsenicum) This combination will treat your runny nose, itchy eyes and sneezing, easing the discomfort of hay fever.

MIXED POLLENS AND GRASSES This mixture of tree, flower and grass pollens helps to desensitize the system against these hay-fever triggers.

NUTRITIONAL ADVICE

Pack your diet with foods that are rich in anti-inflammatory properties to ease congestion, and that are full of vitamin C (a natural anti-histamine). Also, switch from regular tea to green tea, which contains the anti-inflammatory quercetin.

FOODS TO EAT

Foods that are good at helping to relieve the symptoms of hay fever include horseradish, ginger, turmeric, onions, fruit (especially pineapple, berries, grapes, grapefruit and other citrus fruits), vegetables, alfalfa, and nuts and seeds.

FOODS TO AVOID

Avoid dairy products (except plain bio yogurt and cottage cheese) as they are mucus-forming and will worsen symptoms, as well as sugar and refined carbohydrates, which will contribute to any imbalance in your immune system and can in themselves cause inflammation in the body.

right: grasses

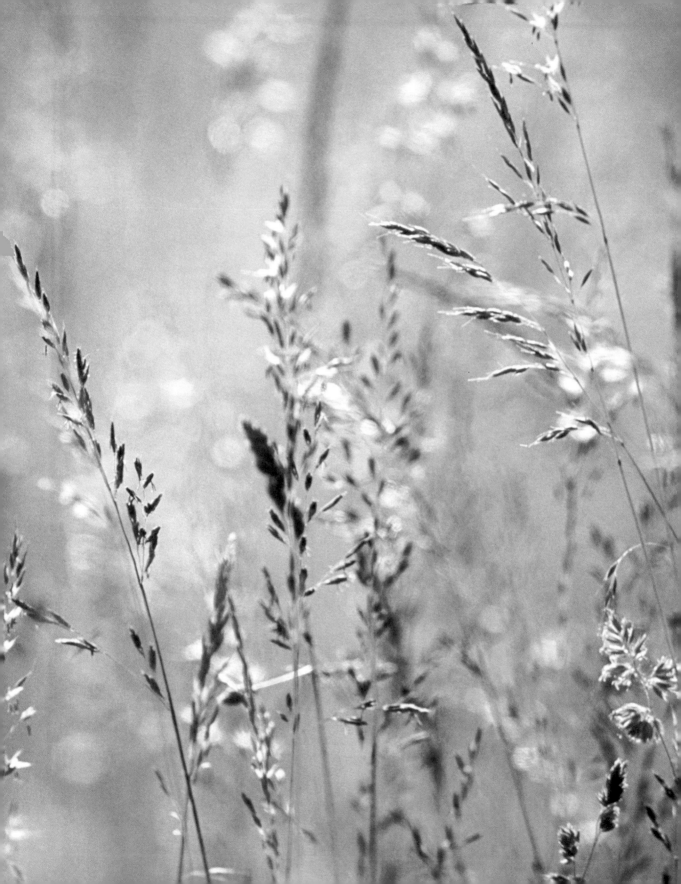

irritable bowel syndrome

IBS affects an estimated one in five people in the US and one in ten in the UK – and always twice as many women as men. Symptoms include stomach cramps and alternating bouts of constipation and diarrhea. In IBS, the gut becomes inflamed – triggered by such things as poor diet, high toxicity, stress and certain medication. This means that it doesn't clear toxins effectively, which leads to further irritation, and so on. Left untreated, IBS can result in problems such as candida, colitis and leaky gut syndrome. The side effects of IBS include bloating, poor skin and tiredness.

The Treatment Program

The single most frequent cause of IBS is toxicity – I have seen as many as seventy to eighty percent of IBS symptoms resolved with a detox. When treating IBS, it is crucial to repair and restore balance to the inflamed gut in order to prevent toxins leaking out of the gut back into the bloodstream (a condition known as leaky gut), and to aim to ensure that the good bowel flora are keeping the bad bowel flora, such as candida, in check.

RECOMMENDED HERBS

The most important aim for an IBS herbal remedy is to care for the gut wall to ease pain and discomfort, and to allow it to repair itself. Take 15 drops each of the following herbal tinctures in a little water or juice three times a day (unless otherwise stated).

ALOE VERA (*Aloe vera*) The juice of this "star" remedy (see pp.106–107) helps to soothe the mucous membranes and reduce inflammation and irritation in the gut wall.
SLIPPERY ELM (*Ulmus fulva*) This herb, taken as a powder mixed with a little water, coats the gut wall, giving it "space" to heal and protecting it from further damage.
LICORICE (*Glycyrrhiza glabra*) Licorice contains the compound glycyrrhizin, which soothes and repairs an irritated gut wall.
PEPPERMINT (*Mentha piperita*) Peppermint relaxes the muscle wall, relieving spasm and pain – although this herb is best avoided during bouts of constipation.

right: licorice (*Glycyrrhiza glabra*)

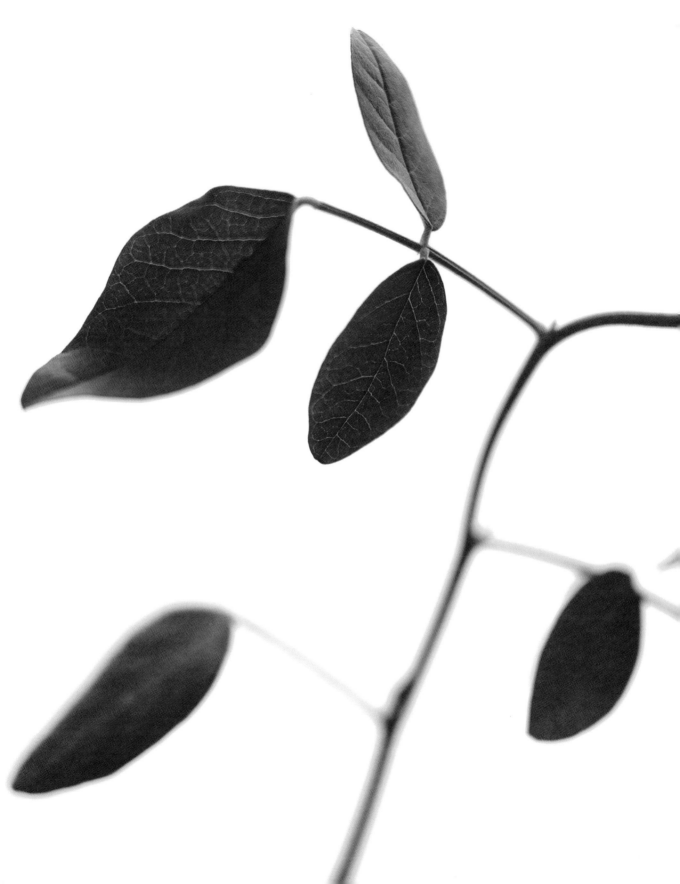

ESSENTIAL SUPPLEMENTS

These supplements will aid the process of detoxification, and also help to repair the gut wall and to balance your gut flora. Take them until your symptoms have gone.

DETOX CAPSULES These capsules contain clay (which binds to toxins to speed their exit from the system), psyllium and apple pectin (which act as gut-cleansers), and L-glutamine and aloe vera (which repair the gut lining).
DOSAGE Three capsules twice daily, morning and night.
ESSENTIAL FATTY ACIDS AND B-COMPLEX VITAMINS This combined supplement provides nutrients that are essential for cell repair to the gut wall.
DOSAGE 1,000mg, daily each morning.

As well as these supplements, be especially vigilant about taking your daily probiotics, as recommended in my daily supplement plan on page 21. Probiotics boost levels of good bacteria in the gut and help to restore the balance of digestive flora.

stress and irritable bowel syndrome

The gut is linked to the brain through a series of nerves and hormonal triggers, which means that feelings such as anxiety and fear can have a significant effect on your gut health. Think about the butterflies you may have felt when you were anxious; or perhaps you had diarrhea when you felt fearful. During the stress response, blood rushes to the legs and arms in readiness for "fight or flight" (see p.112). As blood is diverted away from the gut, digestion slows down, which can contribute to bloating and indigestion. This reaction normally terminates quickly through various feedback mechanisms in the brain. However, if we suffer from prolonged stress, these mechanisms fail and the gut is chronically starved of the blood it needs to work efficiently. If you suffer from IBS, take a look at pages 112–115, and follow the guidelines on how to relieve stress and anxiety, so that you can try to make sure that they are not worsening your condition.

RECOMMENDED HOMEOPATHIC REMEDIES

Homeopathic remedies are wonderful at treating IBS – but ideally you should have a consultation with a homeopath who can prescribe remedies specifically for you. Always do a detox before beginning your IBS homeopathy treatment so that the remedies work as quickly and efficiently as possible. I recommend a combination of the following in a 30c potency up to three times a day as necessary.

CARBO VEG, NUX VOM, LYCOPODIUM These will help with bloating.
ARGENT NIT AND GELSEMIUM If your IBS is accompanied by nervousness, anxiety and nerve-related diarrhea, this combination is great to ease away the stress.

NUTRITIONAL ADVICE

If you have IBS, one of the most important things to remember is not to rush your food – chew it slowly and thoroughly, keeping in mind the thought that digestion begins in your mouth. In addition, steam or lightly cook all you food – raw foods are difficult to digest, while cooked foods are more gentle on an already overloaded gut.

FOODS TO EAT

To aid digestion increase your intake of anti-inflammatory ginger, and foods such as pineapple and papaya, which contain digestive enzymes. Watercress, artichokes, celery, fennel, turmeric and alfalfa help to detoxify your system and so relieve the load on your gut, while linseeds (flax seeds), whole grains, low-fat plain bio yogurt, and fruit and vegetables all generally improve your digestive health.

FOODS TO AVOID

Avoid gas-producing foods, such as pickles, beans, broccoli, legumes, onions, peppers and cabbage, and poor-quality bread. In fact, try cutting out wheat altogether for a while (say, one week), or buy only freshly baked organic sour-dough bread. Gassy drinks are out, too. Sugar in all its forms is the ultimate no-no, as it destroys the balance of good bacteria in the gut; and highly seasoned foods, such as chili, spicy sauces and over-salted foods can irritate the gut, so try to keep them to a minimum.

STAR INGREDIENT: aloe vera

Without doubt, aloe has been one of history's most celebrated medicinal plants. Sumerian clay tablets and Egyptian hieroglyphics document its use more than 3,500 years ago. Amazingly, aloe is actually 96 percent water, and only the remaining four percent contains the compounds that give the plant its miraculous capabilities – as an anti-inflammatory, a healer, a moisturizer and an immune-booster. A desert plant, the leaves store precious moisture, and if they become damaged, special compounds within the plant heal the damage as quickly as possible to minimize moisture-loss. These compounds also protect the plant from attack by fungi and bacteria. There are five species of aloe with therapeutic qualities – aloe vera (also its botanical name) is the most well known.

Understanding Aloe Vera

Aloe vera stores its moisture in a gel in the inner leaves of the plant. Harvesters fillet the leaves to collect the gel, which is then pasteurized and turned into a watery liquid that we can drink as a juice or use to make therapeutic creams and ointments.

The active four percent of aloe contains an impressive 200 or more compounds. In the early twentieth century, Russian opthalmologist Dr Vladimir Filatov (1875–1956) discovered that aloe gel, injected into corneal transplant sites, could work with the body's natural healing mechanisms to regenerate human tissue. Around the same time, in the US medical researchers uncovered the gel's healing properties with regard to sunburn, radiation burn and burns that resulted from fire. More recently, US scientists have shown that certain amino acids in aloe support our body's production of collagen, the protein that gives our skin its elasticity (see p.194); while in Japan researchers have found several enzymes that provide pain relief and scientists in Canada have found anti-viral compounds. Nature's very own cure-all, aloe has failed to gain use in modern conventional medicine only because we aren't yet able to separate its many active compounds.

FOR HEALTH

TO RESTORE GUT DAMAGE Aloe's wound-healing action helps to repair the lining of the gut, making it an ideal treatment for leaky gut syndrome, stomach or peptic ulcers, and IBS, Crohn's disease and ulcerative colitis.

TO DETOXIFY Aloe contains a sugar compound called acemannan that improves the metabolism of the body's cells and so speeds up the process of toxic elimination from them. Its ability to speed the repair of the gut wall also improves detoxification.

TO BOOST IMMUNITY Scientists in the Netherlands have identified two polysaccharides in aloe that stimulate the activity of lymphocytes – immune-boosting white blood cells. Other studies have shown that proteins called lectins in aloe stimulate the immune system specifically to fight tumours.

FOR THE SKIN

TO REDUCE THE SIGNS OF AGING Dr Ivan Danhof at the University of Texas has identified that aloe is able to penetrate the layers of the skin four times faster than water alone. By improving penetration, aloe allows other anti-aging ingredients in skin-care products to act more efficiently. Aloe also promotes anti-aging itself by increasing collagen production, enhancing elasticity, and so making the skin appear more youthful.

TO HEAL SKIN CONDITIONS Whether you suffer from dry skin or acne, oily skin or dandruff, eczema or psoriasis, aloe vera will help to normalize oil production, reduce inflammation, reduce pain and heal wounds. B-vitamins, numerous minerals, and several enzymes and plant sterols work together to give aloe its amazing skin-protective qualities. You can benefit from applying the gel in a topical treatment and from drinking aloe juice. Applying aloe gel to sunburn will help to reduce pain and inflammation, and to repair any damage to your skin.

FIRST AID Aloe has a pain-relieving effect for cuts and grazes and provides antiseptic action by cleansing the open skin. Applying aloe gel after surgery will ensure fast, effective healing and help to reduce scar tissue.

sleep problems

The body needs sleep to repair damage, fight infection and recharge energy. For a few unlucky people, sleep problems – difficulty in getting to sleep, waking frequently through the night and waking up early feeling tired – become a way of life. When these problems are prolonged (chronic), we call the condition insomnia.

The Treatment Program

Depression, anxiety, overtiredness and jetlag are all common causes of sleep problems. Others include overeating, which diverts focus away from sleeping to digesting; and under-drinking, which means that stimulants, hormones and cellular waste build up in the blood rather than being flushed out, leading to aches and headaches. The following program aims to soothe the nervous system and to re-establish a normal sleep cycle.

RECOMMENDED HERBS

Take these herbs, singly or in combination, by mixing 15 drops of each tincture in a little water or juice and taking the mixture once a day at bedtime, for four to six weeks.

OATS (*Avena sativa*) An excellent nerve tonic, oats contain high levels of B-vitamins, and several minerals and other nutrients, which all help restore proper nerve function.
PASSIONFLOWER (*Passiflora incarnata*) Helpful to ease stress and exhaustion, passionflower contains the alkaloid apigenin, which gives it a sedative action.
VALERIAN (*Valeriana officinalis*) Research has shown that valerian is effective at both promoting sleep and improving the quality of sleep. It is particularly suitable if you have fatigue, jetlag or an overactive mind.
SKULLCAP (*Scutellaria lateriflora*) Use this mild sedative if your sleep problems result from worry or an overactive mind, as it contains the flavonoid chrysin (see below).
GERMAN CHAMOMILE (*Matricaria recutita*) This herb contains the flavonoids apigenin and chrysin, which bind to the nerve receptors in the brain that can reduce anxiety and aggression, so calming the body and promoting better sleep.

right: valerian (*Valeriana officinalis*)

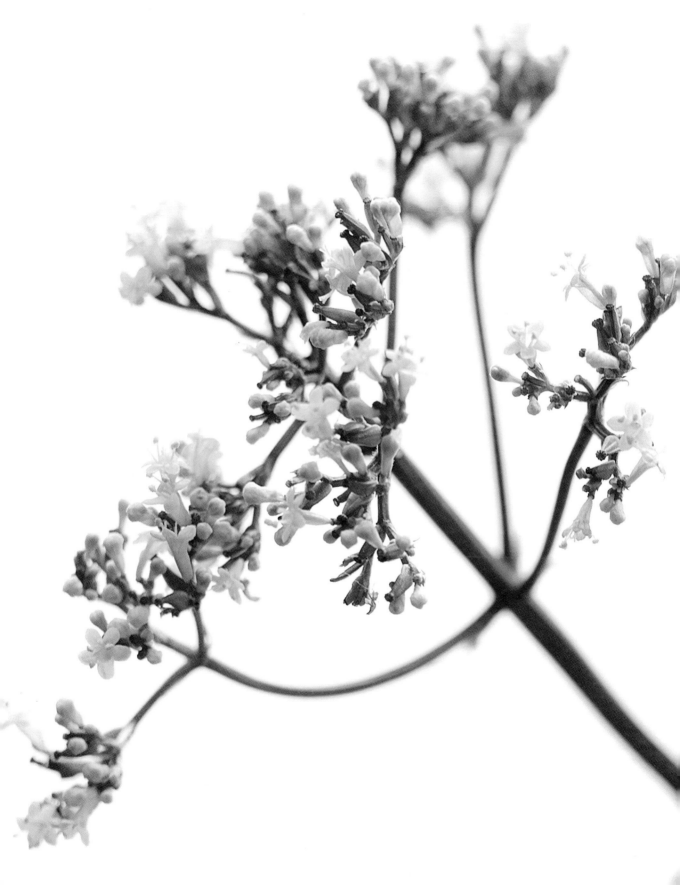

KAVA KAVA (*Piper methysticum*) Kava kava enhances the brain's production of calming chemicals and it may be as effective as conventional medication at helping to relieve sleep problems caused by fear, anxiety or anger.

ESSENTIAL SUPPLEMENTS

Take the following supplements singly or in combination to improve the health of your nervous system and restore overall balance to your mind and body. This is a long-term supplement plan and you can continue taking it on an ongoing basis.

MAGNESIUM AND CALCIUM Calcium is a potent sleep-inducer and both these minerals are necessary for proper nerve function.
DOSAGE 1,000mg daily, taken half an hour before bedtime.
B-COMPLEX VITAMINS Essential for the health of the nervous system, B-vitamins often become depleted during times of stress (the most common cause of insomnia).
DOSAGE As directed on the label.

dealing with snoring

Snoring is a result of the vibration of the soft palate at the back of the roof of the mouth. Any condition that inflames this area – such as the common cold, hay fever, rhinitis, nasal polyps, enlarged adenoids or sinusitis – can cause snoring. The rough, audible sounds and wheezes it produces often lead to a restless night for a sleep partner, but can also disturb the sleep of the snorer themselves. Try the following remedies to see if both snorer and listener can get a better night's sleep.

For the snorer Combine the homeopathic remedies of teucrium marum, hydrastis canadensis and opium in a 6c potency and take two pillules just before bed. This combination will help to reduce inflammation and to clear any accumulated mucus in the nose. Try to sleep on your side, not on your back.

For the listener Take 10 drops oats' tincture in a little water or juice just before bedtime. This will help to relax you and soothe your nerves. Invest in earplugs, too.

RECOMMENDED HOMEOPATHIC REMEDIES

Take all of the following homeopathic remedies in a 6c or 30c potency, just before bed. (If you require help for sleeplessness in children, I recommend visiting a homeopath for a personal consultation, as the reasons for childhood insomnia are so diverse.)

COFFEA Just as coffee causes insomnia, so homeopathic coffea can reduce insomnia, particularly where the causes involve anxiety or an overactive mind.

AVENA SATIVA In a low potency, these homeopathic oats act as a nerve tonic.

VALERIANA Homeopathic valerian helps to relax the nervous system and mind. It is particularly suitable for those unable to take valerian in its herb form (see p.205).

KALI PHOS This excellent nerve tonic is particularly good to treat nervous exhaustion.

NUTRITIONAL ADVICE

Certain foods help to regulate your body's systems, calm your nerves and induce restful sleep, so you should increase them in your diet.

FOODS TO EAT

Foods that contain magnesium, calcium, zinc and B-vitamins will all help to improve the quality of your sleep. These foods include green leafy vegetables (particularly broccoli, kale and cabbage), and nuts and seeds. Like the herbal remedy, rolled oats will act as a great nerve tonic, so try having them for breakfast every day. Milk contains high levels of tryptophan – an amino acid that is a natural sedative – so try the old-fashioned approach of drinking a warm cup of milk before bedtime.

FOODS TO AVOID

Coffee, tea (even green tea), chili and ginger are all stimulants and you should avoid having them in the evening. Among other foods, aubergines (eggplants), tomatoes, courgettes (zucchini), bacon and potatoes all contain tyramine, a natural substance that increases adrenaline production, thus stimulating the body. Try to minimize these foods in your diet if you want to improve the quality of your sleep. Contrary to much popular belief, alcohol disturbs rather than aids sleep, so cut down on your drinking, too.

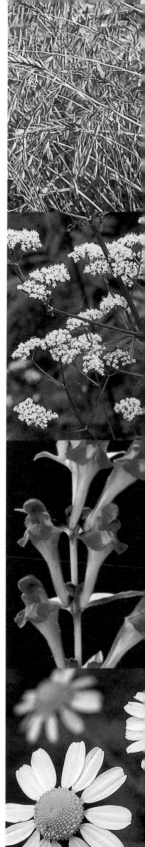

stress

In response to a threat, the body releases a surge of adrenaline (epinephrine), which causes your heart rate to increase, the arteries in your legs to dilate to boost blood-flow to these limbs, and your blood sugar to rise to give you energy. Every available resource in the body diverts to this survival mechanism, enabling you to flee from or fight danger. The adrenal glands also release the hormone cortisol to maintain energy until the danger is over; at which point they secrete the hormone DHEA, which restores calm. This sequence is ideal when danger is real and short-lived. The stress response becomes a problem only when its triggers are prolonged – for example, when a high-pressure job repeatedly initiates the response without giving the body time to recover. This tires out the adrenals and compromises other body systems, in particular the hormone-regulating thyroid and the immune system.

The Treatment Program

Typical symptoms of stress include extreme fatigue, frequent infections, high blood pressure, anxiety, poor digestion, memory loss, mood swings, insomnia and weight gain. In addition, stress can aggravate chronic illnesses such as irritable bowel syndrome (IBS), pre-menstrual syndrome (PMS), and arrhythmia and other heart problems. The treatment program aims to tackle these symptoms, as well as boost your ability to cope with modern stressors. In addition to following the program, identify your stressors and reduce them. Also, make sure you aren't exercising too much, which prolongs the adrenaline response in the body – it's literally physical stress.

RECOMMENDED HERBS

We can divide stress-busting herbs into two groups: nerve tonics, which include oats; and adaptogens, such as rhodiola, which fortify the body's resistance to stress. I recommend you take a nerve tonic together with an adaptogen to get optimum results. The following are my four favourites. Take at least 15 drops of each in a little water or juice, two or three times a day, until you feel balanced and calm again.

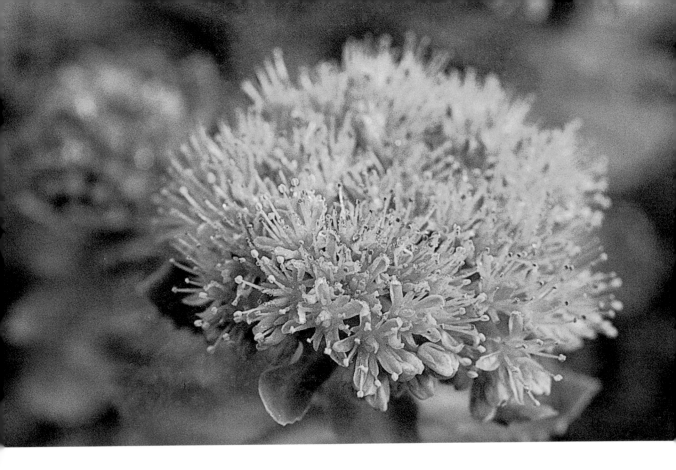

ASHWAGANDA (*Withania somnifera*) This excellent adaptogen helps to reduce levels of anxiety and even the frequency of panic attacks. It is particularly good if your stress is triggered by an excessive workload and you feel deep fatigue.

RHODIOLA (*Rhodiola rosea*) This fantastic adaptogen contains two groups of compounds called rosavins and salidrosides, which studies have shown to be effective in combatting both physical and mental exhaustion resulting from stress.

HOLY BASIL (*Ocimum sanctum*) Also known as tulsi, this tonic reduces cortisol levels and so helps to reduce blood pressure and to balance blood sugar.

OATS (*Avena sativa*) The number-one nerve tonic, oats (particularly the seeds) will help to calm you when you feel overworked, are studying hard or need to recuperate.

ESSENTIAL SUPPLEMENTS

Supplements can help to boost the health of the nervous system and to restore levels of nutrients that become depleted when the body undergoes prolonged stress.

top: rhodiola (*Rhodiola rosea*)

B-COMPLEX VITAMINS B-vitamins have a sedative effect on the nerves and help to maintain the health of the brain's neurotransmitters.

DOSAGE Take as directed on the label.

DETOX CAPSULES Detoxification is important for reducing stress and its effects on the body. It also helps to restore the immune response.

DOSAGE Three capsules, immediately before bedtime.

ESSENTIAL FATTY ACIDS Essential fatty acids are vital to aid the repair and regeneration of neglected cells, and to balance blood-sugar levels, regulating mood.

DOSAGE 1,000mg, daily.

MAGNESIUM AND CALCIUM COMPLEX Stress depletes the levels of these minerals, making supplementation a necessity. Magnesium is essential for adrenal function.

DOSAGE 1,000mg, daily.

As well as these supplements, be especially vigilant about taking your daily antioxidant supplement (see p.21). Antioxidants, especially vitamin C, help to reduce the damage that free radicals cause in the body during stress and to balance the adrenals.

RECOMMENDED HOMEOPATHIC REMEDIES

A tailored course of homeopathy can not only relieve stress, but also teach the body to cope better with the same stressors in the future. The following include a general remedy, and two that are specific to circumstance. Take them as relevant.

KALI PHOS This all-round nerve tonic is an essential remedy of anyone who is stressed, no matter what the symptoms or cause of stress.

POTENCY 6c *DOSAGE* Four pills, three times a day.

NUX VOMICA If your stress makes you prone to outbursts of anger – say, for example, you are prone to road rage – nux vomica will help to calm your temper.

POTENCY 30c *DOSAGE* Two pills, twice daily, morning and evening.

IGNATIA AND NAT MUR This combination is wonderful for calming the constitution of anyone going through a bereavement or loss of some kind.

POTENCY 6c *DOSAGE* One pill up to five times a day.

relaxation techniques

A daily relaxation can help you to release your anxiety and calm your body. The breathing exercise and bathtime ritual on page 45 are perfect. Or, try this simple relaxation at the end of each day. Lie comfortably on your back on the floor. Close your eyes and breathe deeply and steadily. Now tense the muscles in your feet – scrunch up your toes. Hold for a few seconds, then release. Now tense your calves – hold then release; then do the same with your thighs. Continue to tense and release all the muscle groups in this way, all the way up your body, across your shoulders and down your arms. Finish by screwing up your face, then releasing. Feel the tension ebb away with each release. Lie still for a few minutes before you get up.

NUTRITIONAL ADVICE

Without doubt, a great stress-buster is a balanced diet, which will give your body some of the essential nutrients it needs to take care of itself while energy is diverted to calming the stress response. In addition, eat three good meals a day, as well as nutritional snacks inbetween to help control blood-sugar levels.

FOODS TO EAT

Boost your intake of magnesium-rich foods, such as green leafy vegetables, nuts and seeds, and tofu. Whole grains, such as quinoa and brown rice, provide magnesium and B-vitamins, while berry fruits are particularly rich in vitamin C to help to fight off free radicals and improve adrenal function. Oily fish, such as salmon, provide essential fatty acids – although try not to eat them more than twice a week.

FOODS TO AVOID

Steer clear of foods from the deadly nightshade family, including aubergines (eggplants), tomatoes, potatoes and green peppers. These foods contain small amounts of nicotine (as in tobacco), which can accelerate your heartbeat and increase your flow of adrenaline (epinephrine), thus exacerbating the symptoms of stress.

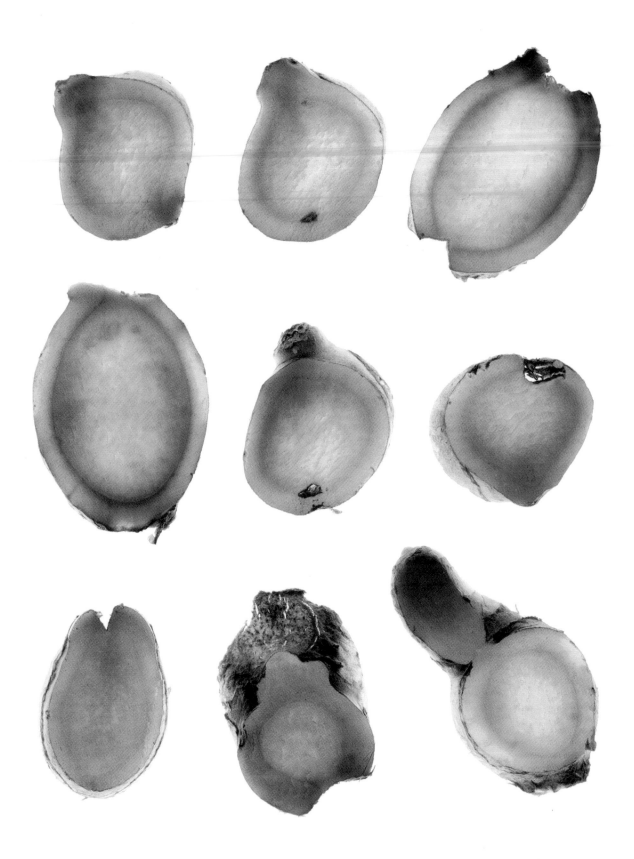

CHAPTER 4

healing aches and pains

Most of us suffer the occasional ache or pain from time to time and, for sportsmen and sportswomen and those with an active lifestyle, the odd knock, bump, scrape or bruise becomes an occupational hazard. However, joint and musculoskeletal pain, such as that in arthritis, is a different story. It can affect any of us at any time and can be extremely debilitating for sufferers, who often live with long-term pain, inflammation and reduced mobility.

Whether you are suffering from joint pain or an injury, the aim of treatment is the same – namely to repair damaged tissue (and neutralize the free radicals that can exacerbate tissue damage) and to reduce inflammation. The overall results are to ease pain and swelling and to speed the healing process, and in the case of arthritis to maximize movement in the affected joints.

The great news is that The Organic Pharmacy's three-pronged approach of using herbs, supplements and homeopathic remedies, together with tailored nutrition, is a highly effective and speedy way to treat these conditions and to achieve these goals. So, if you have a scrape or a bump, or if you have a sports injury, even one that keeps recurring, or if you are suffering from arthritis, dip into this chapter to find natural solutions to your aches and pains.

left: ginger (*Zingiber officinalis*)

arthritis

Arthritis affects more than eight million people in the UK and more than 45 million in the US – and three times more women than men. The two most common forms of arthritis are osteoarthritis (OA) and rheumatoid arthritis (RA). OA is predominantly a wear-and-tear disease – the cartilage between the bones wears away so that the bones themselves start to rub against each other and the joints become painful, swollen and stiff. RA is an auto-immune disease, in which an overactive immune system mistakenly recognizes joint tissue as a foreign pathogen and so attacks the joints, particularly those in the hands, knees and feet, resulting in swollen, stiff and painful joints that may become malformed.

The Treatment Program

Stress, a bacterial, viral or fungal infection in the joint, and an acidic diet can cause tissue breakdown that worsens both forms of arthritis. Furthermore, a diet low in vitamins, minerals and antioxidants and high in toxins can increase the damage in the joints. The following program aims to reduce inflammation and pain, prevent secondary infection, calm the nervous system and improve the diet.

RECOMMENDED HERBS

Herbs will not only ease the pain of arthritis but also reduce inflammation. I suggest you use a combination of three or four of the following herbs. Take 15 drops of the tinctures of each of your chosen herbs in a little water or juice, three times a day for four weeks, and then break for a week before resuming if necessary.

DEVIL'S CLAW (*Harpagophytum procumbens*) This excellent anti-inflammatory helps to reduce pain and increase mobility in joints affected by either OA or RA.
GINGER (*Zingiber officinalis*) Ginger contains compounds called paradol and shogaol. These inhibit the production of certain enzymes (called COX-2 enzymes) that trigger inflammation in the body. The result is a significant reduction in pain and swelling.

BLACK COHOSH (*Cimicifuga racemosa*) Black cohosh contains salicylic acid, which inhibits the COX-2 enzymes (see opposite), helping to reduce inflammation and pain.

WILLOW BARK (*Salix alba*) Similar to aspirin, willow bark eases pain, and because it contains salicylic acid, a COX-2 inhibitor, also reduces inflammation.

BOGBEAN (*Menyanthes trifoliata*) Bogbean contains a bitter agent called meliatine, which is thought to give it its anti-inflammatory effects.

ESSENTIAL SUPPLEMENTS

The following supplements will help to reduce inflammation, repair damaged bone and joint tissue, and strengthen the bones. You can take them on an ongoing basis.

BROMELAIN, VITAMIN (ESTER) C, QUERCETIN COMPLEX Taken together, these three supplements work to reduce inflammation and swelling.
DOSAGE Take this complex as directed on the label.

ESSENTIAL FATTY ACIDS Either in the form of fish oil or linseed (flax seed) oil, essential fatty acids increase the body's production of anti-inflammatory prostaglandins.
DOSAGE 1,000mg, twice daily.

GLUCOSAMINE, CHONDROITIN, MSM COMPLEX This mixture increases the thickness of the fluid in the joints, cushioning the joint and reducing friction pain; and it actively prevents the breakdown of cartilage and helps to rebuild it.
DOSAGE 1,000mg, twice daily.

CALCIUM AND MAGNESIUM This combined supplement will strengthen your bones.
DOSAGE 1,000mg, daily.

In addition to these supplements, be especially vigilant about taking your daily antioxidant supplement (see p.21). Antioxidants help to mop up marauding free radicals, protecting the tissues of the bone from damage.

RECOMMENDED HOMEOPATHIC REMEDIES

I recommend the following homeopathic remedies in a combined pillule at 6c or 30c potency to be taken three times a day for as long as symptoms are present.

CAUSTICUM, RHUS TOX, BRYONIA, GUAIACUM, APIS, FORMICA RUFA This is a wonderful combination of the top six homeopathic remedies that practitioners commonly use to treat both types of arthritis.

NUTRITIONAL ADVICE

Nutrition is a fundamental element in the management of a condition such as arthritis – studies show that by eating the right foods, you can reduce inflammation, fight free radicals and detoxify the body, thus relieving the symptoms and pain of the condition.

FOODS TO EAT

Anti-inflammatory foods include the spices ginger and turmeric (which is also detoxifying), as well as onions, pineapple (which is also detoxifying) and seaweed. Counteract the action of free radicals (see p.195) by eating foods that are rich in

---

two soothing arthritis massage oils

I have found that the following two essential-oil blends are wonderful for relieving sore joints in a topical massage treatment for arthritis. Gently massage the oils into the sore spots and joints, until the oils have been absorbed.

15 drops ginger oil and 5 drops birch oil in 100ml/3½fl oz/scant ½ cup arnica oil I made up this mixture for one of my clients who turned out to be so thrilled with it that I listed the blend as one of our stock products. Arnica is well known for its fantastic soothing action on aching joints, while ginger provides an anti-inflammatory and birch helps to reduce pain.

The Organic Pharmacy's Capsicum and Devil's Claw Cream In this unique The Organic Pharmacy formula, the capsicum and devil's claw cream also contains frankincense and ginger, which all reduce inflammation. I also added some peppermint to act as a local anesthetic, relieving painful nerves and muscles. You can buy it online, or ask a herbalist to make it up for you.

---

antioxidants. Cranberries are especially good, because not only do they contain high amounts of the antioxidant vitamin C, they also help to alkalize the system (acidity worsens arthritis). Sweet potatoes and kiwi fruits are also especially rich in antioxidants. To strengthen the bones and repair damage, boost your intake of alfalfa. Finally, almonds, walnuts, and sesame and pumpkin seeds are all rich in omega-6 and -9 fatty acids, as well as bone-strengthening calcium and magnesium and the antioxidant vitamin E.

FOODS TO AVOID

Steer clear of too much protein (either from meat, or from legumes such as peas, beans and lentils) as these promote acidity in the body – as do salt, soy and vinegar. Foods from the nightshade family (including aubergines (eggplants), tomatoes, peppers and potatoes) contain substances called glycoalkoloids, which may worsen arthritis.

two alkalizing fruit smoothies

Acidity in the body can cause bone tissue to break down, worsening the pain of arthritis. These two smoothies help to alkalize the body.

SMOOTHIE 1
¼ **Cantaloupe melon**
handful fresh cranberries
¼ **lemon**

Place the melon and cranberries in a blender then squeeze the lemon wedge so that its juice is added into the mixture. Whiz in a blender for 2–3 minutes until smooth and enjoy immediately.

SMOOTHIE 2
5 chunks fresh pineapple
flesh of ½ papaya
1cm/½in piece root ginger

Place all the ingredients in a blender and whiz for 2–3 minutes until smooth. Drink immediately. This smoothie is particularly good to alkalize the body and improve digestion after a protein-rich meal.

minor injuries

A minor injury is physical damage to the body such as a wound, fracture, sprain, strain, burn or bruise. The body does several things to protect and heal itself following an injury. First, red blood cells clot to prevent blood loss; then inflammation helps the white blood cells to protect the wound site; and finally new tissue begins to grow to heal the wound.

The Treatment Program

Homeopathy, herbs and certain supplements form an arsenal of remedies that can help at all stages of the healing process – whether the injury is internal or external. Vary the suggestions in this treatment program according to the nature of your injury, the type of wound and the level of pain you experience.

RECOMMENDED HERBS

From the following list of herbal remedies, use those most relevant to your injury.

HERBS FOR INTERNAL AND/OR TOPICAL TREATMENT

KAVA KAVA (*Piper methysticum*) Kava kava is perfect for a muscle injury, as it helps to reduce spasm in the muscle and calm the mind, helping it to deal with pain.
DOSAGE 15 drops tincture in a little water, three times a day for two weeks.
GINGER (*Zingiber officinalis*) A strong anti-inflammatory, ginger inhibits the enzymes that cause inflammation, thus reducing swelling and easing pain. This makes it particularly useful in the treatment of back pain.
DOSAGE 15 drops tincture in a little water or juice, three times a day until the injury has healed or the pain has gone.
GOTU KOLA (*Centella asiatica*) In scientific studies, gotu kola repeatedly reduces inflammation and stimulates collagen synthesis to heal wounds and reduce scarring.
DOSAGE 15 drops tincture in a little water or juice three times a day until the injury has healed; or apply 15 drops tincture mixed into any moisturizing cream.

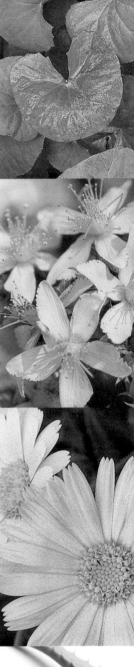

HERBS FOR TOPICAL TREATMENT ONLY

ST JOHN'S WORT (*Hypericum perforatum*) St John's wort is invaluable in the treatment of nerve damage or of wounds at the ends of the toes and fingers, which are rich in nerves. Used topically, it helps to repair tissue and reduce inflammation.
DOSAGE Dilute the tincture in cooled, boiled water (one part tincture to ten parts water). Apply as often as you need. You could apply St John's wort cream, if you prefer.
PROPOLIS (*Resina propoli*) Bees use propolis to protect the hive from bacteria and fungi – and propolis can do exactly the same job for wounds. This star ingredient (see pp.72–73) also stimulates cell regeneration and so is a great wound-healer.
DOSAGE Spray the tincture directly onto small wounds as often as you need.
CALENDULA (*Calendula officinalis*) Excellent for cuts, sores and surgical wounds, calendula helps to stem bleeding and heal wounds. It is antibacterial and antifungal.
DOSAGE Spray the tincture directly onto the wound as often as you need. Alternatively, you can combine the tinctures of calendula, propolis and St John's wort in equal measures to form a spray you can use directly on small cuts, and sores and abrasions. Or use a cream that contains all three and apply as often as necessary to reduce pain and promote wound-healing.
ARNICA (*Arnica montana*) Arnica cream is the best topical preparation for bruises and closed wounds (although never use it on open wounds). Certain components in arnica act to reduce swelling and inflammation; while another component is anticoagulant, and helps to "dissolve" blood clots, making bruises disappear.
DOSAGE Use the cream as often as necessary.
ALOE VERA (*Aloe vera*) Use a good-quality aloe gel or cream to encourage wound-healing and stimulate the growth of new tissue.
DOSAGE Apply as often as necessary.
ROSE-HIP SEED OIL (*Rosa canina*) Apply rose-hip seed oil to scars to promote healing and improve their appearance. This oil is also great for healing radiation burns.
DOSAGE Apply undiluted, twice a day.
DEVIL'S CLAW (*Harpagophytum procumbens*) AND RHUS TOX CREAM This combination will help to ease pain and reduce inflammation in a strain or a sprain.
DOSAGE Apply as often as necessary.

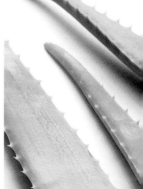

ESSENTIAL SUPPLEMENTS

The following supplement plan will help to repair and regenerate cells, reduce inflammation and heal the skin.

ESSENTIAL FATTY ACIDS These provide the building blocks for the repair and regeneration of cells, as well as inhibiting inflammation and reducing pain.
DOSAGE Two capsules, daily.
ZINC This mineral helps to heal the skin in wounds, and even to prevent scarring.
DOSAGE 15mg, daily.

In addition, be vigilant about taking your daily antioxidant supplement, as recommended on page 21. Antioxidants prevent damage to the body's cells by marauding free radicals (see p.195) and positively promote cell renewal, helping to heal injury.

RECOMMENDED HOMEOPATHIC REMEDIES

The following are the best and most effective homeopathic remedies for treating injuries. Take them in a 6c or 30c potency, four times daily.

CALENDULA, HYPERICUM, ARNICA This combination helps to heal wounds, reduce pain and swelling and aid tissue recovery. It is especially excellent for trauma to nerve-rich areas of the body, such as the fingers and toes, and after dental work or surgery.
RHUS TOX, RUTA, SYMPHYTUM, ARNICA Use this combination if you have a sprain or strain, or ligament damage. It is also ideal if you have a fracture.
ARNICA No household should be without arnica pills. This fantastic homeopathic remedy reduces swelling and bruising and can even help with post-traumatic shock.

NUTRITIONAL ADVICE

All the foods that help the management of arthritis (see pp.120–121) are perfect for supporting the body's work in healing minor injuries because they reduce inflammation and promote healing. In addition, eat organic salmon twice a week. This fish in particular provides proteins that are essential for tissue repair.

right: St John's wort (*Hypericum perforatum*)

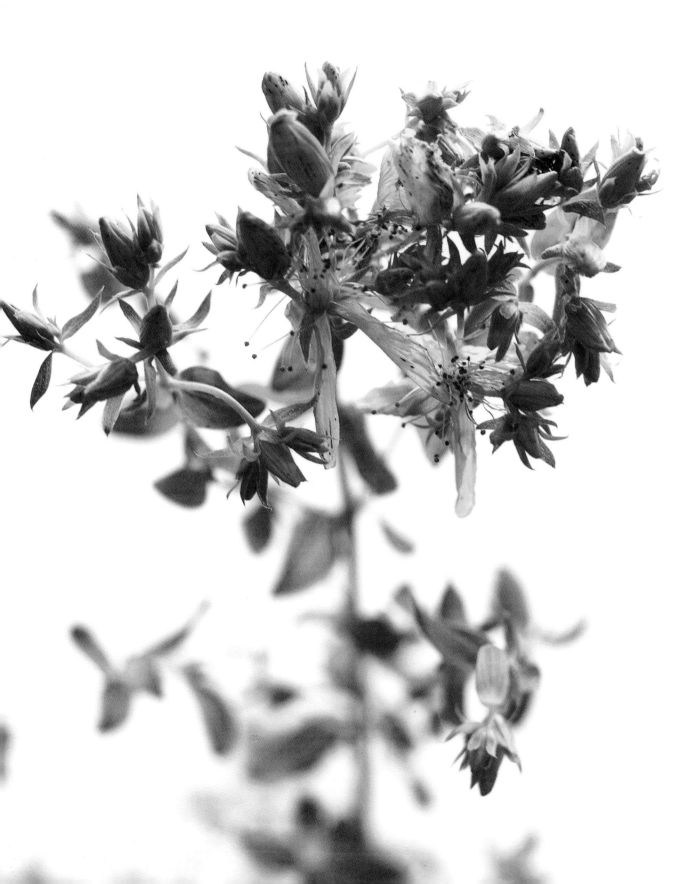

STAR INGREDIENT: calendula

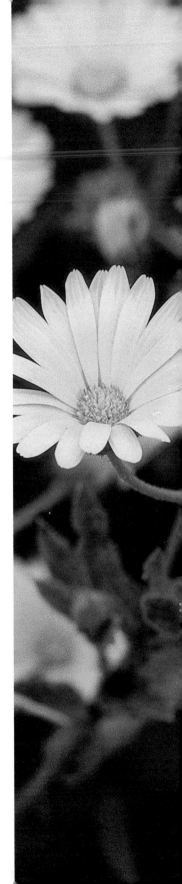

Also known as marigold or pot marigold, calendula (*Calendula officinalis*) was one of the first herbs I learned about while studying homeopathy and I was – and still am – amazed by its medicinal versatility and potency. A Mediterranean plant, its bright yellow–gold flowers, which appear in early summer and continue until the first frosts of winter, are dried and then used in topical ointments, gargles, tinctures and compresses to treat a host of ailments that range from mouth infections to insect bites and sunburn. It also makes a wonderfully calming balm for sore, cracked skin and for cuts.

Understanding Calendula

The flowers of the calendula plant provide myriad therapeutic properties. They contain flavonoids, which are most commonly known for their antioxidant activity, helping to banish free radicals from the body; polysaccharides – a class of carbohydrate that is present in our connective tissues, joint fluid, and cartilage; volatile (essential) oil, which has terpenoid components, thought to be responsible for the flower's anti-inflammatory properties; triterpenes, which help to restore the skin's levels of collagen (see p.194); and carotenoids, which are important antioxidants and give marigold its golden colour.

FOR HEALTH

TO REDUCE INFLAMMATION The triterpenoids and flavonoids in calendula make this herb a wonderful anti-inflammatory. Use it to soothe sore, inflamed and irritated skin conditions and problems, such as cracked skin, sunburn and insect bites.

TO FIGHT INFECTION An excellent antiseptic (it is both antibacterial and antiviral), calendula is wonderful for fighting gum disease and soothing sore throats. For the gums make a mouthwash using 15 drops calendula tincture, 15 drops St John's wort tincture and 10 drops propolis diluted with 10ml (2 tsp) cooled, boiled water. (You should spit out this mouthwash

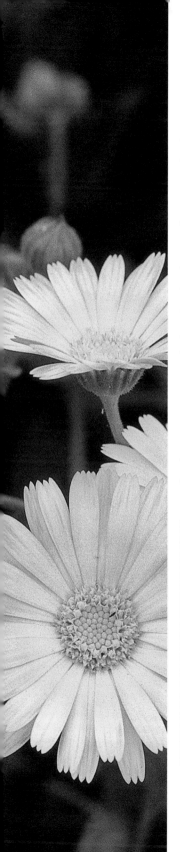

rather than swallow it.) For a sore throat, spray the throat three or four times a day with calendula tincture.

FOR THE SKIN

TO HEAL WOUNDS Applied directly to a cut, sore, ulcer or graze, calendula tincture will help to create new blood vessels and stimulate cell regeneration, which are essential for wound-healing. A healing and disinfecting spray for cuts, sores, ulcers and general abrasions, its ability to stop bleeding in small cuts makes it a perfect post-shaving treatment. As the tincture is alcoholic, it will sting a little when you first apply it – dilute it in a little water for bigger cuts and for children.

If you have had surgery, help your incision site to heal more quickly by combining 15 drops calendula tincture with 15 drops St John's wort tincture and 10 drops propolis. Soak a sterile gauze in the tincture mixture diluted in cooled, boiled water (1 part tincture to 10 parts water) and apply as a compress, twice a day. Once the wound has healed, you can rub in calendula cream instead.

TO REPLENISH THE SKIN With its disinfecting, antibacterial and antiviral activity, I could use calendula in nearly every beauty product I make! It provides the perfect antidote to the ravages of sun, wind, pollution and the effects of stress on the skin.

a medicine from ancient rome

Calendula was given its name by the Romans, who noted that the plants bloomed on the first days – or "calends" – of every month. The ancient Romans used the plant to treat scorpion bites and heal wounds, among many other applications, as well as mixing it with vinegar to season their meat and salad dishes. Calendula blossoms in wine were purported to soothe indigestion, and the petals were used in ointments that cured conditions as diverse as skin irritations, jaundice, sore eyes and toothache. Calendula is often called the marigold, because Roman Catholics once used the flowers in ceremonies to honour the Virgin Mary.

sports injuries

Sports injuries include sprains (a wrenching of a joint, which tears a ligament), aching muscles and muscular strains.

The Treatment Program

While most sports injuries will heal in their own time, supplementation, herbs and homeopathic remedies reduce pain and inflammation, speeding recovery.

RECOMMENDED HERBS

The herbs kava kava and ginger (see p.122) are wonderful for treating the inflammation and pain associated with sports injuries. Use these two as well as the following:

HORSE CHESTNUT (*Aesculus hippocastanum*) Horse chestnut contains a compound called aescin, which helps to reduce bruising and swelling.
DOSAGE Use externally as a cream or massage oil (available from your local herbalist). (You could take the homeopathic form internally at a 6c potency, three times a day.)

ESSENTIAL SUPPLEMENTS

The following supplements will help to repair tissue damage and reduce inflammation.

GLUCOSAMINE, CHONDROITIN, MSM COMPLEX This combination provides three supplements that are vital for the repair of tendons and ligaments.
DOSAGE 1,000mg, three times daily.
CALCIUM, MAGNESIUM, POTASSIUM COMPLEX These minerals help to prevent cramping or muscle spasms and will help to repair damaged tissue.
DOSAGE 1,000mg, twice daily.
ESSENTIAL FATTY ACIDS AND B-COMPLEX VITAMINS This supplement helps the body to produce anti-inflammatory prostaglandins, reducing swelling and pain.
DOSAGE 1,000mg, three times daily.

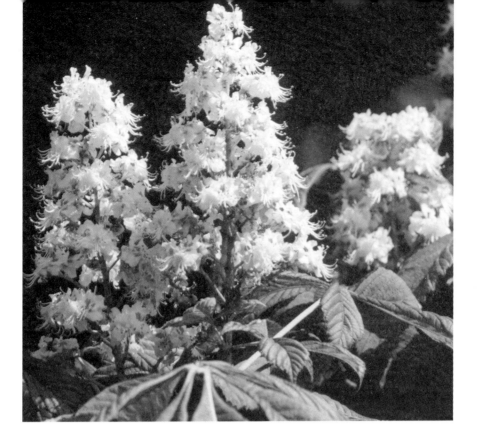

VITAMIN (ESTER) C Vitamin C helps the body to repair torn or damaged tissue.
DOSAGE 500mg, three times daily.

RECOMMENDED HOMEOPATHIC REMEDIES

Take a 30c or 200c potency of each of the following remedies, three or four times a day.

ARNICA As well as taking arnica to treat an injury, try taking it before exercise to help minimize any potential damage.

RHUS TOX, RUTA, SYMPHYTUM, MAG PHOS Take this combination for sprains, strains or ligament damage. I would also recommend it if you have a fracture.

NUTRITIONAL ADVICE

Sports injuries need a diet rich in foods that are anti-inflammatory, reduce free radicals, help to ease pain and swelling, and are good for tissue repair. See arthritis (pp.120–121) for information on foods to eat and to avoid.

top: horse chestnut (*Aesculus hippocastanum*)

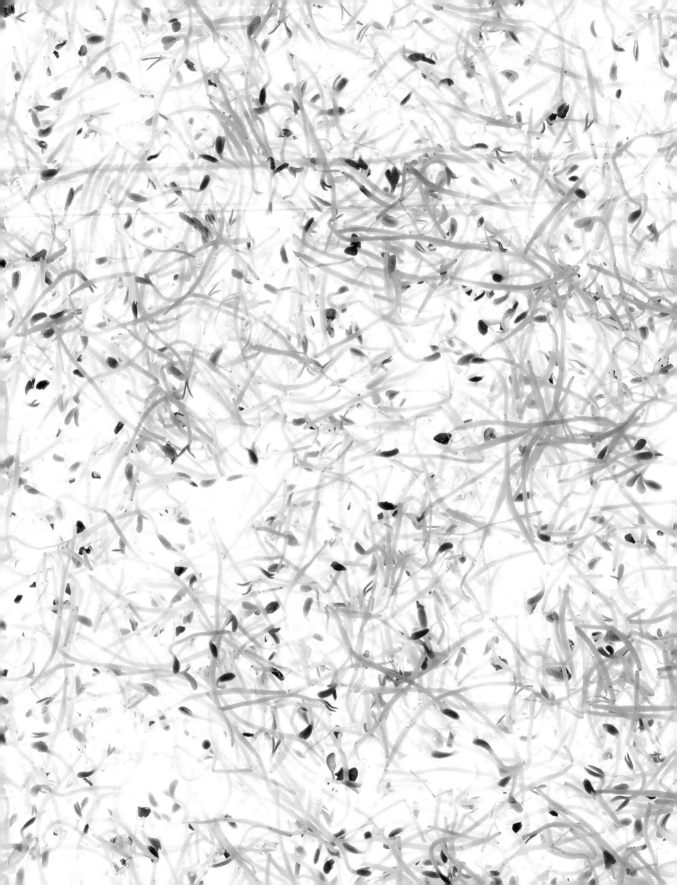

healing the skin

Problems with the skin – from acne to warts – respond exceptionally well to The Organic Pharmacy's three-pronged approach and I am proud to say that I have enjoyed great success in treating almost all skin conditions. As a general rule, the aim when treating skin problems is to boost antioxidant activity in the body in order to reduce the damage by free radicals (which destroy the skin's cells), as well as to aid tissue repair and reduce any inflammation and pain.

Although it may be tempting to think about only topical treatment to tackle skin conditions, it is just as important to treat every condition from the inside, too – remember that your body pushes toxins out through your skin when your other systems of elimination are overloaded (see pp.28–29). The most important thing you can do for any skin condition is to undertake a regular detox to ensure that your body's systems of elimination are working as efficiently as possible, thus reducing the load on your skin. It is also important to consume essential nutrients in order for the skin to repair itself and function properly, and it's crucial to keep stress to a minimum. With these things in mind, the treatment programs in this chapter can help to bring back a healthy glow to your skin – and where necessary restore your confidence, too.

left: alfalfa sprouts (*Medicago sativa*)

acne

The skin produces a natural moisturizer called sebum, which is secreted by the
sebaceous glands in response to hormonal triggers. At certain times, such as during
puberty, the menstrual cycle (for women) and episodes of stress, the body's hormonal
function may become imbalanced. The sebaceous glands then become overactive,
producing an excess of sebum that can block the pores, trapping bacteria and
causing an infection. Acne is the result of this infection.

The Treatment Program

I have treated many cases of acne and there is no simple answer on how to overcome
it. The good news is that a combination of the treatments below, which tackle the
causes and aggravators of acne (hormone imbalance, toxicity, poor immunity, poor
nutrition, constipation and fluctuating blood sugar) help to achieve longlasting results.

RECOMMENDED HERBS

Taken singly or in combination according to your individual symptoms, the following
herbs will help to balance hormones, detoxify the body and boost immunity, and so
reduce the signs of acne. You can take these herbs for eight to 12 weeks, twice a day,
morning and evening. Each dosage is 15 drops of tincture taken in a little water or juice.

RED CLOVER (*Trifolium pratense*) This herb helps to balance the sex hormones,
including testosterone, estrogen and progesterone. It is useful if your acne is brought
on by puberty in girls and boys, or by menstruation or menopause in women.
BURDOCK (*Arctium lappa*) Too much sugar in your system impedes the immune
response and encourages the growth of bacteria. Burdock helps to reduce blood-sugar
levels – and is also antimicrobial and antibiotic.
AGNUS CASTUS (*Vitex agnus castus*) Also known as chaste tree, agnus castus works
on the pituitary gland by helping to balance the hormones. It is especially useful for
acne that worsens just before menstruation.

right: burdock (*Arctium lappa*)

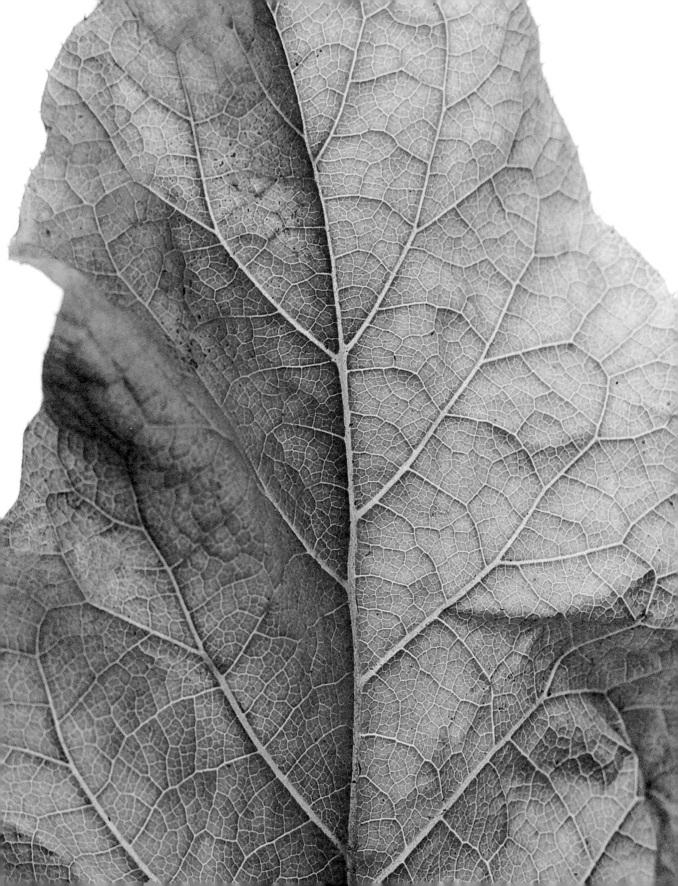

SAW PALMETTO (*Serenoa repens*) This herb helps to prevent the conversion of the male hormone testosterone (which women also have in small amounts) into dihydrotestosterone (DHT), involved in the development of certain types of acne.

YELLOW DOCK (*Rumex crispus*) This herb helps to clear toxins from the system, especially from the blood and the liver. Yellow dock is especially good for pustular acne.

ECHINACEA (*Echinacea purpurea*) If your acne tends to come on during times of illness or otherwise lowered immunity, take this well-known immune-booster.

ESSENTIAL SUPPLEMENTS

In addition to the specific supplements below, during a flare-up of acne, ensure that you take Detox capsules (see pp.46–47), an antioxidant supplement (see p.21), a probiotic (see p.21), and a plant-based multi-vitamin (made up of "green" ingredients, such as spirulina, alfalfa and so on).

ESSENTIAL FATTY ACIDS A deficiency in essential fatty acids is thought to contribute to overactivity in the sebaceous glands, which can lead to acne. Taking this supplement

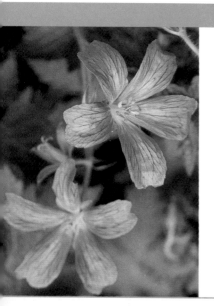

choosing a moisturizer

Most acne sufferers balk at the idea of using oil-based creams on their skin – but oil-free treatments will only dry out the skin forcing the sebaceous glands to produce even more oil, thus worsening the acne. If you have acne, when you buy a facial moisturizer I recommend you opt for products that contain a little oil, as well as some of nature's healers – manuka (which is antibacterial), lavender (antiseptic and healing), tea tree (antibacterial), aloe (healing), cedarwood (balances oil production), rose geranium (antiseptic), propolis (healing and antiseptic) and calendula (healing and disinfecting). Avoid anything that contains parabens (which will disrupt hormone balance) or petrochemicals (which will suffocate the skin).

will help to regulate the activity of these glands.

DOSAGE 1,000mg, twice daily.

EVENING PRIMROSE OIL AND STARFLOWER (BORAGE) OIL These supplements contain gama-linolenic acid, which inhibits the conversion of testosterone to dihydrotestosterone DHT (see Saw Palmetto, opposite).

DOSAGE 500mg, twice daily.

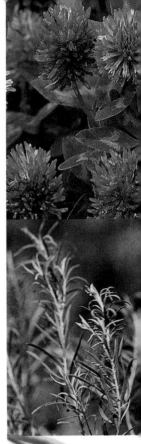

RECOMMENDED HOMEOPATHIC REMEDIES

In general, I don't recommend self-help homeopathic treatment for skin conditions. However, a practitioner may recommend the following remedies (at a 6c potency; one pill twice a day for 14 days), along with the hormonal remedies of either sepia or pulsatilla (see p.159).

SILICA This remedy will push toxins out of the system through the skin – worsening acne at first, but then improving it. It will also help to heal any scarring.

SULPHUR Again, this remedy will detoxify the body through the skin.

KALI BROM Wonderful if you suffer from acne that is characterized by pustules.

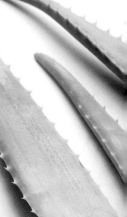

NUTRITIONAL ADVICE

Your diet should aim to boost your intake of antioxidants, as well as variously providing essential fatty acids, antimicrobials and antibiotics. Try to stick to the following guidelines, even when your acne is on the mend.

FOODS TO EAT

Broccoli, carrots, onions, oily fish, nuts and seeds (almonds, walnuts, pumpkin and sesame seeds, and linseeds/flax seeds), watercress, apples, avocados and blueberries are all great for helping the body to recover from acne.

FOODS TO AVOID

Steer clear of the usual culprits – junk foods, alcohol and refined carbohydrates – they provide little nutritional value and will not improve the health of your skin.

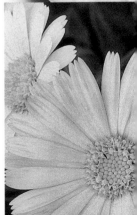

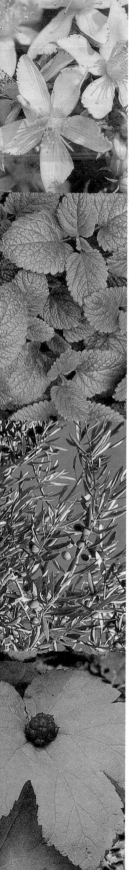

cold sores

Cold sores are caused by the type-1 herpes simplex virus (HSV-1), which invades the cells of the outer layer of the skin (the epidermis), causing fluid-filled blisters. Stress, illness, fatigue, and exposure to the sun, wind or cold are common triggers for a sore.

The Treatment Program

This treatment program aims to beat the cold-sore triggers before they cause an attack, as well as to speed the healing of the cold sore itself.

RECOMMENDED HERBS

At the first tell-tale tingle that a cold sore is coming, take 15 drops of the following tinctures in a little water or juice, five times a day until the cold sore has gone.

ST JOHN'S WORT (*Hypericum perforatum*) This herb (see pp.126–127) is antiviral and also supports the nervous system, making it particularly effective against herpes.
LEMON BALM (*Melissa officinalis*) Lemon balm is both antiviral and calming.
OLIVE LEAF (*Olea europaea*) Compounds in olive leaf are thought to destroy the virus's cell walls. Antioxidants in this herb help to boost the immune system.
GOLDENSEAL (*Hydrastis canadensis*) Antiseptic, anti-inflammatory and astringent, goldenseal helps to dry up the vesicles (blisters) of the cold sore.

ESSENTIAL SUPPLEMENTS

If you are prone to cold sores, I recommend that you take the following supplements as part of your usual daily supplement routine, to help to prevent an attack occurring.

L-LYSINE This amino acid inhibits the virus and reduces the intensity of flare-ups.
DOSAGE 1,000mg, daily.
RED MARINE ALGAE Compounds in red marine algae prevent the virus replicating.
DOSAGE Take as directed on the label.

RECOMMENDED HOMEOPATHIC REMEDIES

Take the following combined homeopathic remedy at a potency of 6c or 30c, three times a day until the cold sore has gone.

NATRUM MURIATICUM AND ARSENICUM ALBUM This remedy combination will help to heal a cold sore quickly (it will also work for genital herpes).

NUTRITIONAL ADVICE

The following advice should help to minimize attacks and speed healing.

FOODS TO EAT

Foods with antiviral nutrients, such as L-lysine, vitamin A, calcium and magnesium, are essential. So, generally eat plenty of fish, chicken, carrots, pumpkins, sweet potatoes, green leafy vegetables, goji berries, shiitake mushrooms, seaweed and alfalfa.

FOODS TO AVOID

Avoid foods that contain high levels of arginine (an amino acid), such as chocolate, peanuts and grains, as arginine intensifies the herpes virus.

cold sore herbal balm

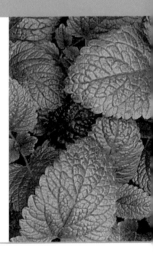

Topical treatments for a cold sore can help fight the viral infection and speed healing. At The Organic Pharmacy we have developed a treatment (called Melissa Complex Balm) that contains of a mixture of antiviral and healing herbs, including lemon balm (sometimes known as melissa, from its Latin name *Melissa officinalis*), propolis, St John's wort and tea tree. Buy it online or ask a herbalist to make it up for you. Studies show that topical application of lemon balm helps reduce the life of a cold sore by forty percent and the addition of propolis and St John's wort speed up healing. Apply the balm as soon as you feel the tingling sensation, and continue to apply it at least five times a day (using a clean finger) until the cold sore has healed.

STAR INGREDIENT: st john's wort

One of the most versatile of my star herbs, St John's wort takes its name because traditionally the plant was harvested on the day in the Christian calender that celebrates the birth of St John the Baptist (June 24). Found growing wild in meadows and gardens throughout North America, Europe and parts of Asia, the herb has distinctive yellow flowers, and leaves that contain small perforations (hence its Latin name *Hypericum perforatum*). Although it is best known for its antiviral and antidepressant properties, St John's wort is also invaluable in the treatment of skin wounds and abrasions.

Understanding St John's Wort

As with all plants, a single component is not responsible for St John's wort's myriad healing effects. Many different constituents give the plant its unique properties. For example, components called hyperforin and hypericin give St John's wort its antidepressant, antibiotic and antiviral effects; several flavonoids in the herb work together to make St John's wort a wonderful wound-healer and anti-inflammatory; and its tannins help to stem bleeding.

FOR HEALTH

TO RELIEVE NERVE PAIN The hyperforin and hypericin in St John's wort make it great for easing all manner of nerve pain – including shingles, toothache, facial neuralgia, back pain and sciatica. For any of these conditions, take St John's wort as a homeopathic remedy (30c or 200c potency, four times a day). If you have had a tooth removed, use the tincture as a mouthwash (dilute one part tincture in ten parts water) every hour after the extraction for up to four or five hours; and for shingles and back pain, also apply St John's wort cream to the affected area.

TO OVERCOME VIRUSES As well as acting on the nerve pain associated with some viral infections, St John's wort has antiviral properties that make it invaluable in the treatment of viral infections such as herpes and the flu. For the duration of the infection, three

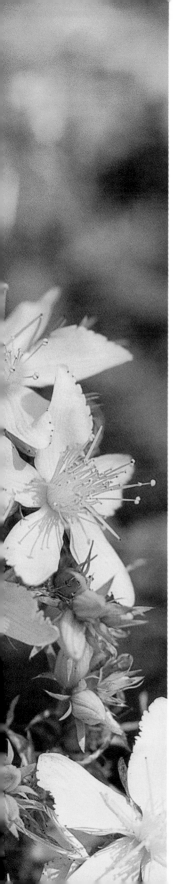

times a day dilute 15 drops St John's wort tincture in a small cup of water and drink. For topical infections, such as genital herpes or cold sores, apply St John's wort cream five times a day until the infection has gone.

Some studies show that the hypericin in St John's wort is particularly effective against retroviruses – a certain group of viruses that often cause tumours.

FOR THE SKIN

TO HEAL WOUNDS The antibacterial and antibiotic properties of St John's wort help to prevent infection and reduce inflammation in wounds, ulcers and sores, as well as promote the growth of new skin cells and strengthen weakened blood capillaries. It also provides a painkiller if the wound is sore. For large wounds, take the herb internally as a homeopathic remedy (30c or 200c potency, three times a day); or wash them with a dilution of one part tincture to ten parts water. For small wounds, such as cuts and grazes, apply a little neat tincture, followed by St John's wort cream.

An alternative for cuts and ulcers is a first-aid spray treatment made by combining equal measures of the tinctures of calendula, St John's wort and propolis. The spray is antiseptic, will stop or slow down bleeding, relieve pain and promote healing.

TO HEAL BURNS As a burn heals, a grainy tissue (known as granulation tissue) covers the surface of the burn to protect it from infection and allow new skin to grow underneath. Studies show that St John's wort speeds up the growth of the granulation tissue and repairs damaged skin three times faster than conventional burn treatments. St John's wort will also help to prevent scarring. Apply a St John's wort cream to the burn four or five times a day until healing is complete.

FOR THE MIND AND EMOTIONS

TO IMPROVE MOOD Scientists are uncertain how St John's wort works to improve mood, but one hypothesis is that the herb prevents the transmission of certain mood hormones into the brain. Well known for its anti-depressant action, St John's wort is also excellent for seasonal affective disorder and anxiety. Take 15 drops of St John's wort tincture in a small amount of water three times a day.

eczema (dermatitis)

An inflammatory reaction in the skin, eczema is characterized by blister-like bumps, swelling, crusting and, in extreme cases, thickening and scaling of the skin. The condition has many triggers – including leaky gut syndrome, gut-flora imbalance and synthetic perfumes – but is most often caused by an overactive immune system.

The Treatment Program

All too often conventional treatments for eczema tackle only the symptoms of the condition, rather than the cause. The aim of my program is also to heal and soothe the skin (and you can use many of the treatments topically, making them a safe alternative to steroids) – but then I strongly recommend that you visit a homeopath who will give you a tailored treatment that aims to resolve your eczema at its roots.

RECOMMENDED HERBS

Take each of the following herbs at a dosage of 15 drops of tincture in a small amount of water or juice, three times a day for at least eight weeks. If after this time you can see no improvement, seek the advice of a homeopath or homeopathic pharmacist.

CHICKWEED (*Stellaria media*) Chickweed contains certain natural detergents, called saponins, that calm and soothe the skin, helping to reduce itching. You can also use chickweed topically in the form of a cream (apply six times a day to affected areas).

GERMAN CHAMOMILE (*Matricaria recutita*) When the immune system over-reacts to cause eczema, the body releases histamine, which exacerbates inflammation. German chamomile has antiallergic and anti-inflammatory properties that calm the skin. You can also apply it as a cream (at least twice a day to affected areas).

NEEM (*Azadirachta indica*) Neem contains compounds called nimbin (which calms the skin) and nimbidin (which is anti-inflammatory). It is antibacterial and antifungal, and so protects broken skin from secondary infection, and it is healing. You can also use it topically as a cream (at least twice a day to affected areas).

WILD PANSY (*Viola tricolor*) Used to heal skin complaints for hundreds of years, the wild pansy helps to reduce inflammation and itching in the skin.

ESSENTIAL SUPPLEMENTS

The following supplements help to cleanse the body, reduce inflammation and fortify and heal the skin.

DETOX CAPSULES A body overloaded with toxins will push impurities out through the skin, causing or worsening eczema, so regular detox is essential for eczema sufferers.
DOSAGE Three capsules, taken at night.

EVENING PRIMROSE OIL AND BORAGE OIL These oils contain gamma-linolenic acid (GLA) and linoleic acid, which are converted in the body to anti-inflammatory prostaglandins. The oils will also help to lubricate and nourish the skin.
DOSAGE 500mg, twice a day; or apply externally as a cream, twice a day.

LINSEED OIL Linseed (or flax seed) contains compounds that the body turns into prostaglandins, which help to reduce inflammation.
DOSAGE One tablespoon, daily.

PROBIOTICS Although the exact mode of action still eludes us, research shows that taking probiotics can help to improve eczema.
DOSAGE Two billion, twice daily.

In addition, try to be especially vigilant about taking your daily antioxidant supplement (see p.21), as not only does this wonder-supplement reduce inflammation, it also helps your skin tissue to repair and heal.

RECOMMENDED HOMEOPATHIC REMEDIES

For longlasting relief, see a homeopath, who can tailor a treatment to your history and symptoms. The following will calm an attack. Use a 6c potency, three times a day.

GRAPHITES, ARSENICUM, PETROLEUM These three remedies will help to ease the typical symptoms of eczema, such as open, weepy skin that is irritated and itchy.

treating childhood eczema

Eczema is most commonly a condition that begins in childhood. There are three essential remedies to try for childhood eczema, given in two ways.

Internal treatment On a daily basis give your child two billion probiotics, which are available in powder form and so can be added to water, juice, yogurt or milk. Add to this a teaspoon of linseed (flax seed) oil. It is essential to see a homeopath for internal homeopathic treatment.

Topical treatment Use The Organic Pharmacy's Ultra-dry Skin Cream to soothe itching and help to heal sore skin. Buy online or ask a herbalist to make it up for you.

NUTRITIONAL ADVICE

In many cases tailoring your diet to gain optimal nutrient intake provides a key to longlasting relief from eczema. A food diary can help to identify which, if any, foods worsen your condition so that you can avoid them. Every day, make a note of everything you eat, and also of any symptoms you experience.

FOODS TO EAT

Foods that are anti-inflammatory, such as pineapple and the spice turmeric, help to soothe the skin and reduce itching. Also effective are foods that have an anti-histamine action, including ginger and foods rich in vitamin C, such as kiwi fruits and all yellow, orange and red fruits and vegetables. Too much acidity in the body will worsen the condition – try to eat plenty of alkaline foods, such as avocados, grapefruits and spinach (see also p.15).

FOODS TO AVOID

Avoid foods that cause too much acidity in the body, such as salty foods, soy and vinegar, as well as allergens, such as artificial colourings and preservatives, and hydrogenated fats. Also avoid anything that your food diary reveals may be an eczema trigger – wheat and dairy are common culprits.

right: evening primrose (*Oenothera fruiticosa*)

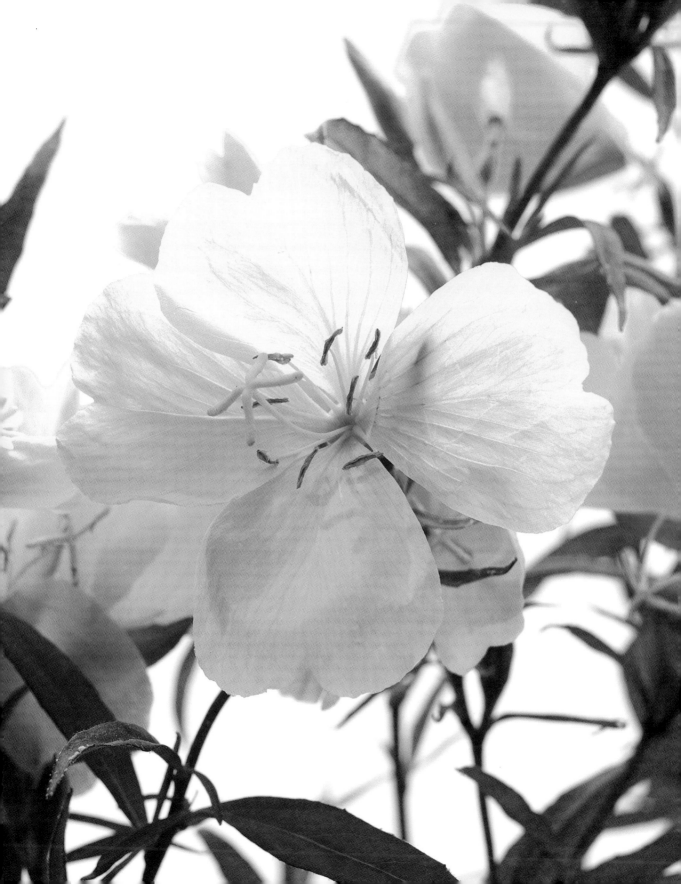

psoriasis

In healthy skin new skin cells form in the lowest layers and, as they age, migrate upward until they reach the skin's uppermost layer – a process that takes around 28 days. An auto-immune disorder, psoriasis quickens the cell-aging process so that, instead of taking 28 days, it takes only around eight. Typically, this results in increased numbers of blood vessels in the skin, causing inflammation and angry red patches that have a silvery-white, scaly appearance. In extreme cases, psoriasis can also affect the nails, causing pitting and thickening.

The Treatment Program

We still don't know for certain why the immune system reacts to cause psoriasis, but we do know that toxicity, stress, poor immunity, lack of sunlight, bacterial infection, oxidative stress (a harmful by-product of oxygenation in the body), and poor nutrition all seem to worsen the condition. The treatment program tackles these triggers.

RECOMMENDED HERBS

The following herbs help to reduce the symptoms of inflammation, redness and irritation, as well as reduce triggers and balance the immune system. Take 15 drops of the tinctures of the following herbs three times a day for at least two months. After two months take a break for two weeks, and then resume if necessary.

LYCIUM (*Lycium barbarum*) Also known as goji, lycium is rich in the vitamins beta-carotene, C, B1 and B2. It also contains the anti-inflammatory agent beta-sitosterol, as well as linoleic acid (an essential fatty acid), and a polysaccharide that appears to boost the immune system. As well as taking it internally, you can apply lycium to affected areas of skin in the form of a cream (twice a day).

NEEM (*Azadirachta indica*) Clinical studies have shown that in cases of psoriasis, neem can reduce inflammation and help to heal the skin. You can use it internally, or apply it externally as a cream (twice a day, combined with lycium cream if possible).

WILD PANSY (*Viola tricolor*) Compounds in wild pansy have an anti-inflammatory effect on the skin. You can take it internally, or apply it as a cream (twice daily).

OREGON GRAPE (*Mahonia aquifolium*) Oregon grape has been shown to soothe and heal the skin in more than seventy percent of a test group of sufferers. Its main constituents are thought to inhibit oxidative stress in the body. You can apply this herb as a cream (twice daily), as well as taking it internally.

SARSAPARILLA (*Smilax regelii*) Flavonoids in sarsaparilla help to regulate the immune response, making this remedy perfect for treating auto-immune conditions such as psoriasis. The flavonoids also cleanse the liver, which makes sarsaparilla a good detoxifier, too.

ESSENTIAL SUPPLEMENTS

As with eczema, the aim of taking supplements to treat psoriasis, in conjunction with homeopathic remedies and herbs, is to reduce inflammation and toxin levels, to lubricate the skin, and to ensure a good supply of antioxidants. For these reasons, you can follow the same supplement regime given for eczema (see p.139).

RECOMMENDED HOMEOPATHIC REMEDIES

During a flair-up of psoriasis, the following remedy combination will help to control your symptoms. For long-term relief, consult a homeopath for a program tailored to your unique constitution and medical history. Take this remedy in a 6c potency, twice a day.

GRAPHITES, ARSENICUM, BERBERIS AQUEFOLIUM, PETROLEUM This combination is designed to work on the skin and kidneys to help reduce inflammation.

NUTRITIONAL ADVICE

If you suffer from psoriasis you need to stock up on the anti-inflammatory, anti-histamine and alkaline foods that help to soothe and balance your skin and system. All the good foods listed in eczema (see p.140) are great to eat if you suffer from psoriasis, too. All the foods to avoid if you suffer from eczema will also worsen psoriasis – so check out the list and ban them from your diet.

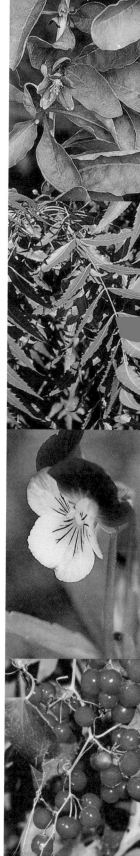

rosacea

An inflammatory skin condition, rosacea is characterized by redness – as a result of dilated blood vessels – on the cheeks, nose, chin or forehead.

The Treatment Program

The following will help to reduce the triggers and relieve the symptoms of rosacea.

RECOMMENDED HERBS

Take 15 drops of each of the following herbal tinctures in a little water or juice up to three times a day, for two to three months (unless otherwise stated).

PINE BARK EXTRACT (*Pinus maritima*) Pine bark extract inhibits pro-inflammatory enzymes in the body, so reducing redness and inflammation on the skin.

BILBERRY (*Vaccinium myrtillus*) The tannins in bilberry make this herb a potent astringent – helping to open dilated blood vessels. Use for only two weeks at a time.

RED CLOVER (*Trifolium pratense*) This purifier helps to clear toxic waste from the body.

MILK THISTLE (*Silybum marianum*) Milk thistle's active ingredient, silamarin, helps cleanse the liver, and it also has antioxidant and anti-inflammatory properties.

skin creams to treat rosacea

As rosacea is a topical condition, I find topical treatments (in conjunction with internal treatments) are wonderfully effective. Buy online or ask a herbalist to make up for you a cream containing bilberry, pine bark extract, aloe vera and tamanu. Used for centuries by South-Sea islanders to treat skin conditions, tamanu oil contains a non-steroidal anti-inflammatory agent called calophyllolide, a unique fatty acid called calophyllic acid, and other natural anti-inflammatory compounds called coumarins. All of these properties enable this lovely oil to help heal, repair and calm the skin.

ESSENTIAL SUPPLEMENTS

Take the following supplements to support your body and help reduce bouts of rosacea. You can take the supplements on an ongoing basis.

DETOX CAPSULES Toxicity – particularly of hormonal waste – "heats up" the body from the inside. Taking detox capsules will support the liver in its hormone-balancing work.
DOSAGE Three capsules at night for twenty days.
ESSENTIAL FATTY ACIDS EFAs will help to reduce chronic inflammation.
DOSAGE Two capsules daily, or as directed on the label.
ANTIOXIDANTS These will help to protect the skin cells from free-radical damage.
DOSAGE Two capsules, twice daily.
ASTAXANTHIN A potent anti-inflammatory that protects cells from oxidative stress.
DOSAGE Take as directed on the label.

RECOMMENDED HOMEOPATHIC REMEDIES

Take the following remedy in a 6c potency twice a day to control your symptoms.

BELLADONNA, FERRUM PHOS, ARSENICUM These remedies help to reduce the symptoms of redness and inflammation.

NUTRITIONAL ADVICE

As well as eating foods that improve the health of your skin (see p.191–193), the following should ease the symptoms of rosacea. Keep a food diary, too (see p.140).

FOODS TO EAT

Boost your intake of anti-inflammatory foods such as ginger, alkalizers such as cranberry and melon, and detoxifying foods such as alfalfa and seaweed.

FOODS TO AVOID

A US survey of rosacea sufferers identified hot spices as common triggers, as well as alcohol, hot drinks, chocolate, tomatoes, citrus fruits and wine (particularly red wine).

scarring

When the skin's surface breaks open, the collagen fibres in its connective tissues extend to form a scar. By reducing inflammation you can reduce visible scarring.

The Treatment Program

Whatever the cause of a scar, you can use a number of remedies both topically and internally to improve the formation of connective tissue (boosting the circulation helps with this) – sometimes reducing the appearance of even old, established scars.

---

creams and oils for scarring

Combine the following topical treatments with the internal program. Apply each cream or oil two or three times a day.

Rose-hip seed oil This essential skin-healer contains eight different antioxidants, including beta-carotene, lycopene and vitamin C, which help to reduce inflammation and curb free radicals. It also contains the anti-inflammatory quercetin and essential fatty acids (which keep the skin supple). It has been clinically proven to help all kinds of scars, resulting from injury, radiotherapy and burns. Try to find a good-quality oil that has a deep orange (not yellow) colour.

Tamanu oil This oil's non-steroidal, anti-inflammatory ingredient calophyllolide and a unique fatty acid called calophyllic acid make it wonderful in the treatment and healing of scarring.

Aloe vera cream or gel A combination of more than 200 active constituents gives aloe is anti-inflammatory and skin-healing properties (see pp.106–107).

Calendula, St John's wort and propolis cream The combination of these three wound-healing herbs is perfect to help minimize or reduce scarring. You can even apply the combination to an open wound.

RECOMMENDED HERBS

Take 15 drops of each tincture in water or juice, three times a day for four to six weeks.

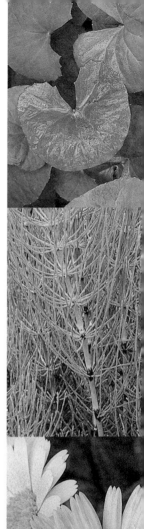

GOTU KOLA (*Centella asiatica*) Gotu kola contains triterpene, which tests have shown to be effective at reducing both new and old scarring.

HORSETAIL (*Equisetum arvense*) Horsetail is the richest of all plants in a component called silica, which is the raw material required for collagen formation.

ESSENTIAL SUPPLEMENTS

These supplements provide nutrients essential for tissue repair and reducing swelling.

CALCIUM, MAGNESIUM, POTASSIUM COMPLEX This combined supplement is made up of nutrients that are essential for proper cell function.
DOSAGE Take as directed on the label.

ESSENTIAL FATTY ACIDS AND VITAMIN-B COMPLEX These nutrients will help to reduce inflammation in healing skin.
DOSAGE Take as directed on the label.

ANTIOXIDANTS These will reduce inflammation.
DOSAGE Two capsules, twice daily.

RECOMMENDED HOMEOPATHIC REMEDIES

For post-operative scarring, take these remedies at a 200c potency, three or four times a day. For all other types of scarring, take a 6c potency, three times a day.

ARNICA, ST JOHN'S WORT, CALENDULA These are a "must" for post-surgery wounds.
THIOSINIMUM, SILICA, GRAPHITES, CALC FLUOR This combination is both an excellent scarring preventative and will help to reduce old scars, too.

NUTRITIONAL ADVICE

The nutritional advice that I gave for arthritis (see p.120) is also perfect to help prevent scarring, as it reduces inflammation and promotes healing.

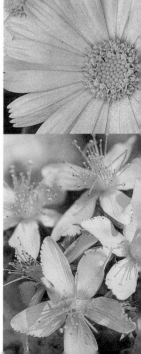

STAR INGREDIENT: rose-hip seed oil

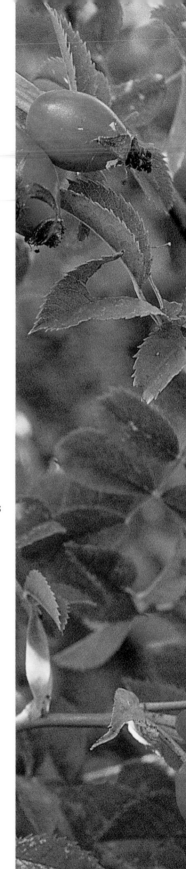

High up in the Andes mountains in Chile grows a beautiful wild rose, the bright red fruits (hips) of which contain seeds that are rich in an oil that has remarkable healing properties. I first came across this oil more than a decade ago when I received a sample from Chile. From past experience, I was expecting a pale yellow colour and a slightly fishy smell – but I was pleasantly suprised. This was a rich orange–red oil with a fresh, clean smell. It was virgin cold-pressed to give a purer quality rose-hip seed oil that was soon to amaze me with its wonderful ability to repair the skin.

Understanding Rose-hip Seed Oil

At the University of Concepción in Chile, researchers have carried out studies to assess the action of rose-hip seed oil on scarring caused by severe accidents, burns, ulcers, acne, and irradiated skin. The researchers applied the oil to volunteers twice a day for several months. Their findings were amazing. The oil was effective at keeping fresh scars to a minimum, and also helped to heal scars that were up to twenty years old. Its action on healing the skin and reversing damage caused by the sun, radiotherapy and chronic ulcers was nothing short of remarkable. Further testing on sun-damaged skin, pigmentation, and acne scarring gave increasingly great results: rose-hip seed oil eradicated sun damage, brown spots and wrinkles and removed all signs of acne scars.

Rose hip's astonishing abilities have shown themselves in other studies, too. Dr Hans Harbst, head of radiology at the Chilean Airforce Hospital, found that when applied to skin damage caused by radiotherapy, rose hip enabled lesions to heal faster than with no oil at all, and that there were fewer scars.

All these qualities are the result of three active constituents in

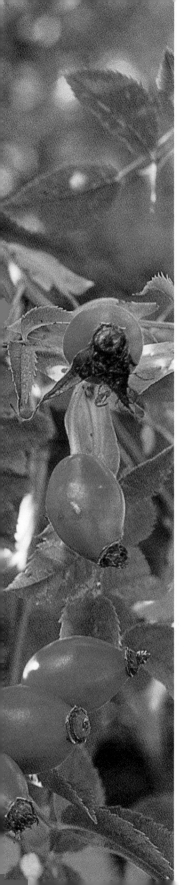

rose-hip seed oil. The first is the group of abundant essential fatty acids that help to maintain the health of cell membranes and regenerate and rejuvenate skin tissue. Second, rose-hip seed oil contains trans retinoic acid – a form of vitamin A that is the natural precursor to retinoic acid, which is found in many topical skin-care creams. Whereas synthetic retinoic acid may cause side effects such as dryness, trans retinoic acid works together with the other components of rose-hip seed oil to reduce wrinkles and restore elasticity – with no side effects whatsoever. The final group of active constituents is antioxidants. Two of these, quercetin and iso quercetin, inhibit the activity of the enzyme responsible for the breakdown of elastin (see p.194), thereby increasing the elasticity of the skin. In addition, research shows that quercetin can help to reduce the formation of keloid and hypertrophic scarring (raised, overgrown and discoloured scars).

FOR THE SKIN

TO REDUCE SCARRING Whether your scarring is a result of acne, chicken pox or surgery, rose-hip seed oil will help to promote healing and prevent scar formation. Use two drops undiluted on the wound twice a day.

TO REDUCE THE APPEARANCE OF STRETCH MARKS Perfectly safe to use during pregnancy, rose-hip seed oil will help to improve the appearance of old stretch marks, as well as easing away the new. Rub a little of the undiluted oil into your marks twice a day.

TO SOOTHE SUN-DAMAGED SKIN The action of rose-hip seed oil on sun-damaged skin is beyond doubt. The oil reverses sun damage, and protects the skin from UVB radiation. (But never use it as a substitute for suncream.) Apply it undiluted to patches of sun-damaged skin once a day.

TO REDUCE WRINKLES AND PIGMENTATION The same qualities that enable this oil to protect the skin from sun damage, ease away wrinkles and pigmentation. Anti-inflammatory properties and antioxidants offer protection from free radicals.

TO IMPROVE ELASTICITY The high essential-fatty-acid content of rose-hip seed oil make it wonderful for keeping the skin supple and young-looking. Apply the undiluted oil twice a day, in the morning and evening.

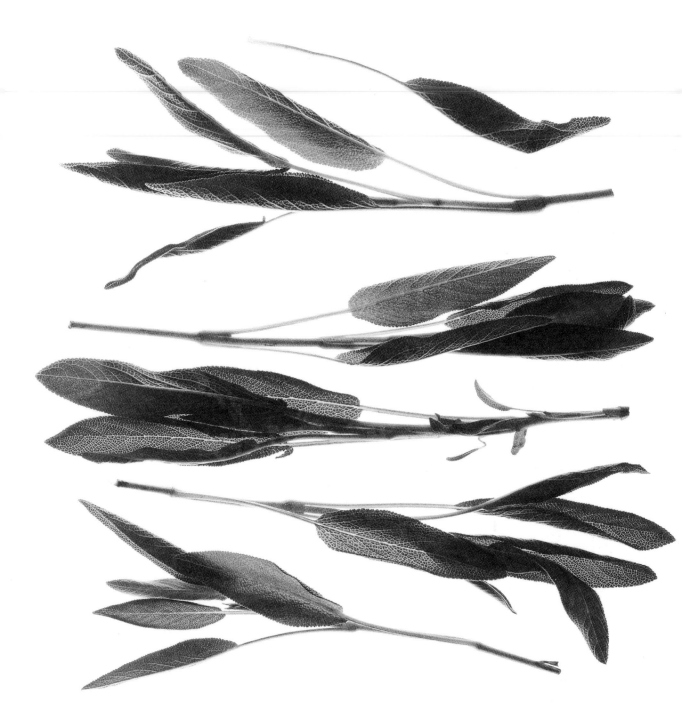

CHAPTER 6

healing women's problems

Man or woman, we each have a unique genetic make-up. This means that each of us is prone to a unique set of health problems. However, the complex female body, which includes all the apparatus that enables us to bear children, means that, in my view, "women's problems" need a special section all of their own. Although every woman is unique, the underlying causes of women's problems are often very similar. With the exception of cystitis, which tends to be caused by an infection, a hormonal imbalance is usually at the root of conditions that are specific to women – irregular periods, premenstrual syndrome and menopause among them. Fertility is also reliant on the hormones – although, of course, this isn't necessarily a condition that occurs only in the female body, which is why this chapter includes remedies that boost male reproductive health, too.

In this chapter I've presented you with a wonderful arsenal of herbs and homeopathic remedies, supported by supplements and nutritional advice, that will help to bring your hormones into balance naturally and without side effects. And don't forget detox! The build-up of stale hormones in the body is a primary cause of toxicity – which then goes on to cause imbalance in all the body's systems, including in the amazingly complex reproductive system.

left: sage (*Salvia officinalis*)

cystitis

If bacteria in the bladder multiply faster than we expel them in the urine, they may attach themselves to the walls of the urinary tract causing cystitis. The infection is characterized by a frequent need to pass urine, which will often burn or sting.

The Treatment Program

Natural medicine provides many remedies for cystitis. Although the ultimate cause is bacterial, weakened immunity, vigorous intercourse, high sugar in the urine and the absence of bacteria-fighting enzymes in vaginal secretions can all trigger attacks.

RECOMMENDED HERBS

Some herbs are anti-microbial to destroy bacteria; others are diuretic; still others soothe the mucous membranes of the urinary tract. Take 15 drops of these tinctures in a little water or juice every hour for the first day, and then five times on the second day, four times on the third day, then three times a day for the following week.

GOLDENSEAL (*Hydrastis canadensis*) This herb is antiseptic and anti-inflammatory, and its astringent properties help to clear mucus and congestion in the urinary tract.
ECHINACEA (*Echinacea purpurea*) Echinacea reduces inflammation in the bladder, stimulates immunity and attacks bacteria.

the importance of water

Dehydration can exacerbate cystitis. If you're prone to attacks, make sure you drink at least six glasses of filtered water every day. Then, during an attack, increase your water intake to 12 glasses (think of it as one an hour until you've drunk the 12). In this way, you will help your system to flush out the bacteria that cause the infection and speed your recovery.

UVA URSI (*Arctostaphylos uva ursi*) Anti-microbial and disinfecting, uva ursi fights *E coli* (bowel bacteria) and is a diuretic. It is effective only if the urine is alkali (see below).

ESSENTIAL SUPPLEMENTS

CRANBERRY Unsweetened cranberry juice contains compounds that help to prevent bacteria from sticking to the walls of the urinary tract.
DOSAGE Take as directed on the label.
CALCIUM, MAGNESIUM, POTASSIUM COMPLEX This combination of nutrients will help to calm an irritated bladder and replenish lost stocks of potassium.
DOSAGE Take as directed on the label.

RECOMMENDED HOMEOPATHIC REMEDIES

Take the following combination of remedies every hour during an attack, preferably in a 30c potency. Reduce the frequency as your symptoms improve.

BERBERIS, STAPHISAGRIA, APIS, CATHARIS, EQUISETUM, CAUSTICUM All these homeopathic remedies support the work of the bladder and ease the burning sensation during urination.

NUTRITIONAL ADVICE

The following nutritional advice aims to boost your intake of foods that improve the health of your bladder and fight infection, and minimize those that won't.

FOODS TO EAT

Eat plenty of antibacterial and antiseptic foods, such as garlic, as well as diuretic foods – watercress, celery, parsley and cucumber. Ginger will help to reduce inflammation.

FOODS TO AVOID

Avoid anything that irritates the bladder or dehydrates the body – coffee and tea in particular. Foods and drinks that encourage bacterial growth are also out: avoid fruit juices, especially citrus juices, and all sugary foods and drinks.

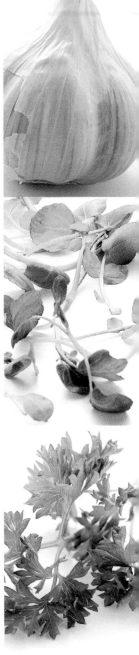

irregular periods

Usually lasting around 28 days, the menstrual cycle charts the movement of an egg from an ovary to the womb. In readiness to receive a fertilized egg, the womb develops a thick lining. However, if the egg is not fertilized, the womb sheds its lining, resulting in a period. The regularity of your menstrual cycle depends upon the balance of your reproductive hormones, which trigger this process.

The Treatment Program

This treatment program focuses largely on hormone balance, because any imbalance, at any point in the cycle, can cause irregular periods.

RECOMMENDED HERBS

Take 15 drops of each of the following herbal tinctures in a little water or juice twice a day for eight weeks (or longer if under the supervision of a practitioner).

AGNUS CASTUS (*Vitex agnus castus*) This A1 hormone-balancer acts on the pituitary gland to regulate hormone levels in the ovaries.
FALSE UNICORN ROOT (*Chamaelirium luteum*) Hormone-like saponins in this herb have a balancing effect on estrogen and progesterone levels.

ESSENTIAL SUPPLEMENTS

The following supplements help to balance the whole system and the hormones.

DETOX CAPSULES A detox is vital to repair the body and to get all the systems, including the reproductive system, working efficiently again.
DOSAGE Three capsules twice a day for ten days.
ESSENTIAL FATTY ACIDS AND B-COMPLEX VITAMINS Omega-3 essential fatty acids are essential for good hormone health; the B-complex will fortify you against stress.
DOSAGE Two capsules, daily.

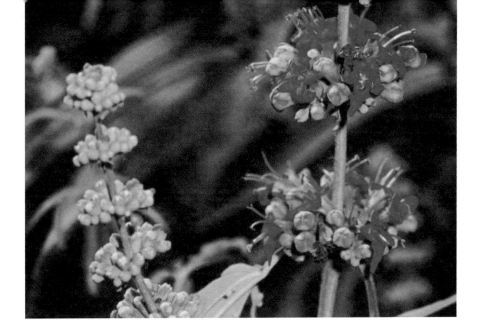

ADDITIONAL SUPPLEMENTS

Take these supplements according to the causes of your condition:

• antioxidants (if you suffer from endometriosis or polycystic ovarian syndrome; two capsules, daily) • multi-vitamin (if you have a nutritional deficiency; as directed on the label) • magnesium and calcium complex (if you are stressed; as directed on the label).

RECOMMENDED HOMEOPATHIC REMEDIES

If your irregular periods are caused by emotional trauma, it's vital that you see a registered homeopath for a consultation. In all other cases, the following remedies can help. They will continue to work long after you have stopped taking them.

SEPIA, KALI CARB, PULSATILLA, CAULOPHYLLUM Take two pillules of this combination, in a 6c potency, twice daily for two to three weeks.

FRAXINUS AMERICANA Take five drops of this remedy in a 6x potency, morning and night, to reduce fibroids. You can take fraxinus americana in the long term if necessary.

NUTRITIONAL ADVICE

Organic foods are especially important if you suffer from irregular periods, as pesticides and herbicides can cause xenoestrogens (environmental chemicals with estrogen-like activity) to accumulate in the body. For all other nutritional advice, see Infertility (p.163).

top: agnus castus (*Vitex agnus castus*)

premenstrual syndrome

US research suggests that almost forty percent of women aged between 14 and fifty experience some symptoms of PMS, while research in the UK puts this figure at ninety percent for British women. Symptoms include anxiety, irritability, abdominal bloating, backache, breast swelling and tenderness, sweet cravings, acne, water retention, mood swings and, in extreme cases, depression, confusion and insomnia.

The Treatment Program

This program aims to balance your estrogen levels, correct any imbalance of serotonin and dopamine in the brain, or of calcium and magnesium in the body (usually because of stress), and balance low blood sugar, which can all exacerbate PMS.

RECOMMENDED HERBS

Take 15 drops of each of the following herbal tinctures in a little water or juice twice a day for the 12 days before your period is due.

AGNUS CASTUS (*Vitex agnus castus*) This is the number-one herb for PMS symptoms, particularly breast tenderness, irritability, bloating and sweet cravings.
SKULLCAP (*Scutellaria lateriflora*) Great for PMS characterized by problems such as irritability, mood swings and anxiety, skullcap also helps to relieve cramping.
DANDELION (*Taraxacum officinale*) The phytosterols in dandelion have a diuretic action that relieves symptoms such as bloating. It also helps to cleanse the liver.

ESSENTIAL SUPPLEMENTS

In addition to tackling PMS, these supplements may also help to relieve period pain.

MAGNESIUM, CALCIUM, B6 COMPLEX High levels of the hormone prolactin (which can lead to mood swings and even depression) can result from a deficiency in magnesium and vitamin B6. The combination is also excellent in the relief of cramps and contains calcium to replenish stores that may be depleted by excess estrogen.

DOSAGE As directed on the label.

ZINC Again, low levels of zinc can encourage the release of prolactin (see above).

DOSAGE 15mg, daily.

DETOX CAPSULES These help to cleanse the body and, in particular, the liver.

DOSAGE Three capsules at night.

STARFLOWER OIL OR EVENING PRIMROSE OIL Both these oils are rich in gamma-linolenic acid (GLA). Research shows that a deficiency in GLA may contribute to symptoms of PMS.

DOSAGE 1,000mg, daily.

RECOMMENDED HOMEOPATHIC REMEDIES

I have found the following combinations to be extremely effective against PMS and its symptoms. Take them four times a day in a 6c or 30c potency while your symptoms last.

SEPIA, NUX VOM, PULSATILLA This combination is particularly helpful if your PMS is characterized by the symptoms of irritability, sadness, anger and weepiness.

CHAMOMILLA, DIOSCOREA, COLOCYNTHIS, MAG PHOS These remedies help to relieve pain and cramping during your period.

NUTRITIONAL ADVICE

In general, make sure you avoid the steroids and hormones used in farming by eating organic produce, and drink bottled water to avoid the estrogens in tapwater.

FOODS TO EAT

Eat plenty of essential fatty acids, as in oily fish and walnuts (which are also rich in zinc, calcium and magnesium). Other mineral-rich foods include pumpkin and sesame seeds and green leafy vegetables, barley and brown rice.

FOODS TO AVOID

Keep away from junk foods, as these upset your chemical balance.

infertility

More than five million couples in the US and around 3.5 million in the UK are thought to have difficulty conceiving – although many will become pregnant in time. Doctors use the label "infertile" only after a couple has been unsuccessful for more than a year, or if a woman is consistently unable to carry a pregnancy to term.

The Treatment Program

At around the middle of a woman's menstrual cycle, a surge of hormones triggers an ovary to release an egg, which travels down the Fallopian tube to meet a sperm. Once fertilized, the egg implants in the lining of the uterus, after which the woman must produce various hormones, such as progesterone and human chorionic gonadotropin (HCG), to create a conducive environment in which the fertilized egg can develop safely. Anything that interferes with any one of these vital steps – including the health of the sperm – can result in infertility. My program aims to bring everything into balance for both partners to optimize a couple's chances of conceiving.

RECOMMENDED HERBS

For women, the following herbs will regulate menstruation, balance hormones and provide a uterine tonic that will help to prevent miscarriage. The men's herbs will help to optimize sperm count, motility and health. Ask your pharmacist or herbalist to mix each combination in equal quantities. Take 15 drops of the relevant herbal mixture three times a day. Stop taking the combinations once you are pregnant.

FOR WOMEN

FO-TI (*Polygonium multiflorim*) An ancient Chinese herb, fo-ti promotes female libido and research has shown that it increases female fertility.

FALSE UNICORN ROOT (*Chamaelirium luteum*) This herb has an adaptogenic or balancing effect on the female sex hormones, and it is thought to help infertility that is caused by a lack of follicle stimulating hormone (FSH), which triggers egg-release.

MACA (*Lepidium meyenii*) Studies of this Peruvian root show that maca helps to stimulate the ovarian follicles, where a developing egg matures.

AGNUS CASTUS (*Vitex agnus castus*) This hormonal wonder-herb normalizes the action of the pituitary gland, which is responsible for the release of FSH.

SAW PALMETTO (*Serenoa repens*) Saw palmetto can help to reduce cases of infertility caused by polycystic ovarian syndrome (see box, below).

SHATAVARI ROOT (*Asparagus racemosus*) This reproductive tonic contains steroidal saponins that may reduce uterine spasms, which may help to prevent miscarriage.

WILD YAM (*Dioscorea villosa*) By converting to progesterone in the body, this herb can help to correct imbalances in a woman's levels of progesterone and estrogen.

FOR MEN

SAW PALMETTO (*Serenoa repens*) This herb acts on the male hormone testosterone and is thought to increase sperm production. It is also used to improve general testicular health.

ASTRAGALUS (*Astragalus membranaceus*) Clinical trials indicate that astragalus has a stimulating effect on sperm production and helps to improve sperm motility.

MACA (*Lepidium meyenii*) Used to improve egg development in women, maca can enhance sexual function in men (and women) and increase sperm production.

FO-TI (*Polygonium multiflorim*) Also used to promote female libido, fo-ti will increase male sexual energy and help to improve the quality of a man's sperm.

OATS (*Avena sativa*) A well-established nerve tonic, oats are particularly useful where stress and nervous exhaustion are major causes of male infertility.

treating polycystic ovarian syndrome

In PCOS cysts form on the ovaries, often resulting in reduced fertility. The herb saw palmetto contains fatty acids and phytosterols that act on the sex hormones and this may be why this particular herb seems to be so effective at treating the symptoms of PCOS. Take 15 drops of the tincture in a little water or juice, three times a day.

ESSENTIAL SUPPLEMENTS

Both partners should take the following supplements while trying to conceive.

DETOX CAPSULES A clean body provides an environment that is more likely to support conception – just as a seed is more likely to survive and grow better in clean soil!
DOSAGE Take three capsules, morning and evening. Drink eight glasses of water during the day.

STARFLOWER OIL OR EVENING PRIMROSE OIL These are both rich in gamma-linolenic acid (GLA), which in women helps to balance the hormones, and in men may help with sperm motility. Both these oils also help you to cope with stress.
DOSAGE 1,000mg, daily.

ZINC, CHROMIUM, SELENIUM COMPLEX These minerals are vital for healthy sperm production. Chromium deficiency is associated with low sperm count and selenium deficiency is associated with poor sperm motility. Zinc also encourages cell renewal and repair, which may be especially helpful if the woman suffers from endometriosis.
DOSAGE As directed on the label.

B-COMPLEX VITAMINS INCLUDING FOLIC ACID The B-vitamins help to keep all your organs healthy and enable your body to cope better with stress. The body uses folic acid (also a B-vitamin) to make new cells.
DOSAGE As directed on the label.

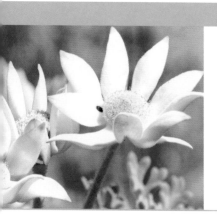

australian bush flower essences

Bush flower essences harness the healing properties of flowers that are found in the Australian bush to restore the balance between mind and body. I recommend the following if you are trying to conceive. Take 7 drops morning and evening directly on your tongue.

For women She oak, which will help to clear blocked emotions.

For men Flannel flower, which will help to promote intimacy.

VITAMIN (ESTER) C This important vitamin helps to protect developing cells and, in men, helps to keep sperm mobile.
DOSAGE 1,000mg, twice daily.

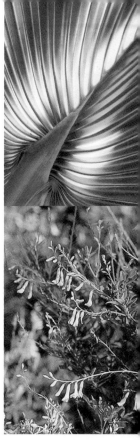

RECOMMENDED HOMEOPATHIC REMEDIES
The following combination of remedies is useful for women if miscarriage is a common symptom of infertility. Take a 6c potency twice a day for two to three weeks as soon as you know you are pregnant. (For all other kinds of infertility, please have a personal consultation with a homeopath, as an individualized program for both of you is vital.)

CAULOPHYLLUM, CIMICIFUGA, SEPIA, SABINA Ask your pharmacist to make this blend, which combines several of the major female remedies.

NUTRITIONAL ADVICE
For cases of infertility, organic food, particularly organic meat, which helps to keep the body free from artificial hormones, is more important than ever – a medical requirement, if you like. The following applies to both men and women, unless I've noted otherwise.

FOODS TO EAT
As well as eating plenty of fresh, organic fruits and vegetables, both of you should try to increase your intake of foods rich in B-vitamins, zinc, manganese and selenium (whole grains are a good example). Cook with and drink only filtered or bottled water so that you avoid all the toxins (and especially the estrogens) in tapwater, which may upset your delicate hormonal balance and so impair fertility. Men should boost their intake of zinc-rich shellfish.

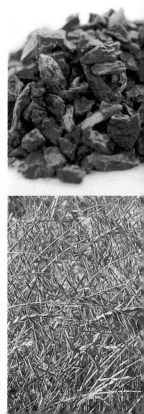

FOODS TO AVOID
Hydrogenated fats (found in processed and fried foods) reduce fertility in both men and women, so take special care to avoid them. Also, be aware that studies have shown that licorice can decrease testosterone levels in men, leading to sexual dysfunction. Both partners should avoid alcohol.

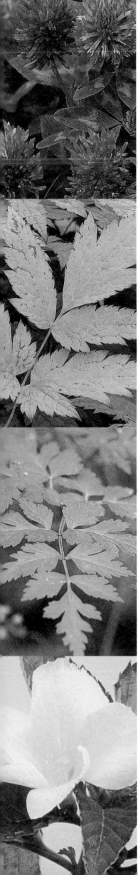

menopause

A normal part of a woman's cycle of life that usually occurs between the ages of 45 and 55, menopause begins when falling levels of the sex hormones estrogen, progesterone and testosterone in the woman's body mean that her ovaries stop working, her reproductive system closes down and monthly menstruation ceases. Her hormone levels may begin to fall off gradually – sometimes from as early as 30 years of age – as her body prepares for menopause. This lead-up to menopause is called perimenopause.

The Treatment Program

Hot flashes; night sweats; sleep disturbances; anxiety, depression and mood swings; weight gain; lost libido; weakened bones, muscles and skin-tone; breast cysts; and vaginal dryness are all symptoms of menopause. The following program contains remedies that aim to regulate hormone levels to ease all these symptoms, as well as remedies that target specific problems, such as lost bone density and low libido.

RECOMMENDED HERBS

Take the following herbs singly or in combination as 15 drops of each tincture in a small amount of water or juice, twice a day for as long as necessary.

RED CLOVER (*Trifolium pratense*) Rich in estrogen-like compounds, red clover can reduce the frequency of hot flashes, help to increase bone density, and discourage the growth of benign breast cysts (the opposite effect of many synthetic estrogens!).
BLACK COHOSH (*Cimicifuga recemosa*) This herb is known for its ability to reduce night sweats, hot flashes, vaginal dryness and insomnia.
DONG QUAI (*Angelica sinensis*) This herb sensitizes the estrogen-receptor sites, encouraging their uptake of estrogen from the blood.
DAMIANA (*Turnera diffusa*) Damiana helps to boost libido, which may fall as the levels of sex hormones fall, and ease menopause-related depression and anxiety.

MACA (*Lepidium meyenii*) This Peruvian herb regulates the glands responsible for producing hormones, and so balances estrogen, progesterone and testosterone levels. Additionally, it enhances libido (in both men and women).

SAGE (*Salvia officinalis*) Studies show that sage can reduce problem sweating (such as night sweats and hot flashes) by up to fifty percent.

ESSENTIAL SUPPLEMENTS

Take these supplements as soon as you notice the first signs of menopause.

MAGNESIUM AND VITAMIN B6 COMPLEX Boosting magnesium and B6 helps reduce levels of the hormone prolactin in the body, which at high levels can suppress ovulation.
DOSAGE 500mg magnesium daily; 10mg B6 daily.

CALCIUM It's important to supplement calcium during menopause, as falling levels of estrogen interfere with the body's ability to absorb this nutrient.
DOSAGE 1,000mg calcium, daily.

STARFLOWER OIL OR EVENING PRIMROSE OIL Both these oils are rich in a substance called gamma linolenic acid (GLA), which produces anti-inflammatory, hormone-like substances that include prostaglandins. These help to keep the skin smooth and supple (as well as having beneficial effects on heart health).
DOSAGE 1,000mg, daily.

DETOX CAPSULES The body needs to function optimally to keep the symptoms of menopause to a minimum. Detox also helps to maintain the skin's elasticity.
DOSAGE Three capsules every night during your ten-day detox and for ten further nights immediately following on from it.

woman essence

Known simply as "Woman essence", this Australian bush flower essence (see p.162) helps to support the hormonal system, relieving symptoms of menopause and improving mood. Take 7 drops, morning and evening, directly on your tongue.

RECOMMENDED HOMEOPATHIC REMEDIES

I have achieved excellent results controlling menopausal symptoms such as hot flashes, irritability and insomnia by prescribing the following combinations of homeopathic remedies. Take them in a 6c potency, twice a day, ongoing.

PULSATILLA, SANGUINARIA, SEPIA, LACHESIS, APIS MEL, OOPHORINUM Ask your pharmacy to make this blend, which combines several of the major female remedies.

NUTRITIONAL ADVICE

From boosting nutrients to help with bone density to regulating hormones, the world of food offers us many opportunities to ease this important time in a woman's life.

FOODS TO EAT

Research suggests that diets rich in plant-derived phytoestrogens, particularly from legumes and foods such as fennel, celery and parsley, may help to modulate the body's hormonal fluctuations at the time of menopause. Soy is well known as an estrogen regulator, as its phytoestrogens block the uptake of aggressive forms of the hormone that can cause imbalances. However, eat soy only infrequently (or choose the fermented varieties of tofu or miso), as it can interfere with protein metabolism and thyroid function. (If you have had breast cancer, avoid soy products altogether, but stock up on linseeds/flax seeds, which contain lignans and may help to prevent breast cancer.) Try to eat foods that will protect your bone density – these include salmon or other oily fish that are rich in essential fatty acids; calcium-rich foods such as dairy; as well as green leafy vegetables, whole grains and sesame seeds, which supply other vital nutrients, including magnesium. Finally, always use olive oil, as it is rich in vitamin E and so can help to reduce hot flashes and vaginal dryness.

FOODS TO AVOID

All women approaching or going through menopause should avoid junk, fatty and stimulant foods. In particular, be aware that carbonated drinks will strip your body of calcium, contributing to the weakening of your bones.

right: sage (*Salvia officinalis*)

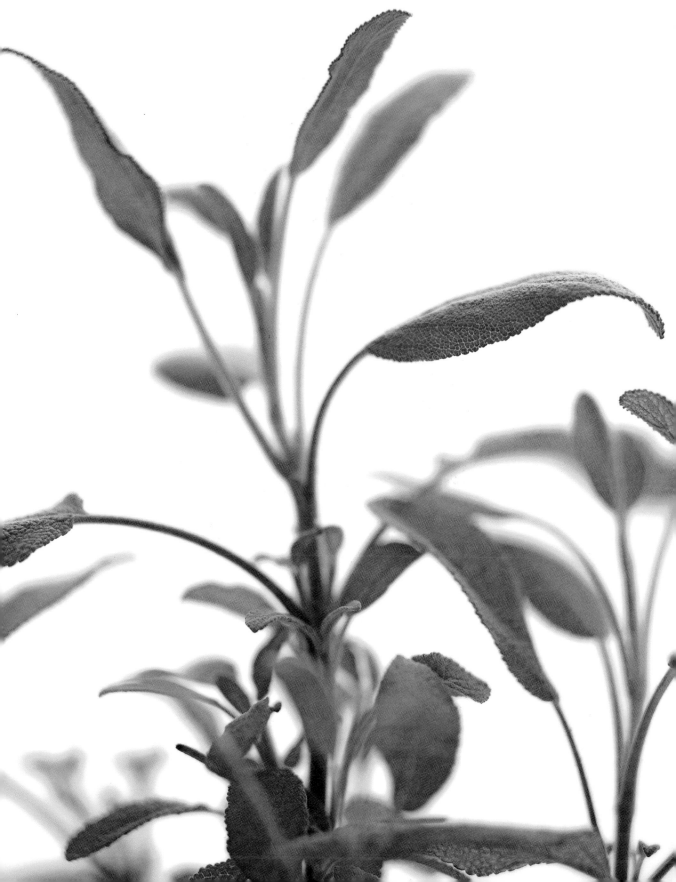

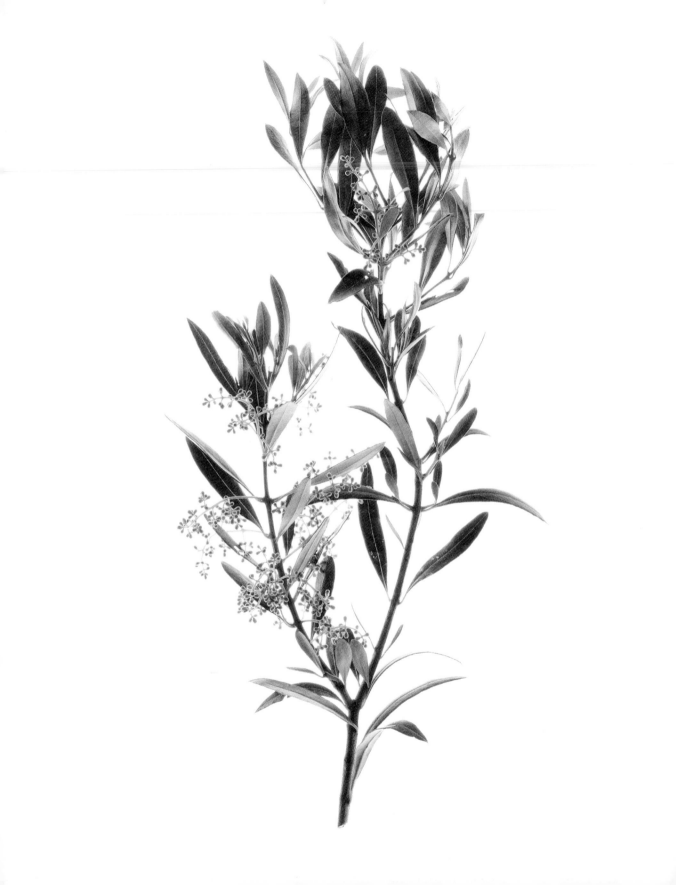

CHAPTER 7

treating childhood illnesses

Every parent knows that happy, healthy, sociable children frequently pick up bugs. However, many of us agonize over how best to treat these frequent infections. Increasingly, parents are wary of giving their children antibiotics and other conventional medicines, and yet many mothers I know also feel a little uncertain about treating their children with herbal remedies and homeopathy – even when they are happy to treat themselves this way! All I can say is that, as a mother of two, I have first-hand experience of the safe, natural and effective treatments that the worlds of herbs and homeopathy can provide for your children. In fact, because their little systems are purer and less toxic than grown-up systems, children often respond to homeopathic remedies better than adults. However, one thing I would generally never recommend for children is detox. If your child is fed a good, balanced and nutritious diet that comprises only the best fresh, organic produce, he or she should never need to undergo a cleanse.

The conditions in this chapter are those that I am most commonly asked to treat at The Organic Pharmacy – and they include conditions as diverse as teething and chicken pox. When you need to use a plan, look at the age advice carefully before you begin. Remember, in the case of illness, if your child's symptoms persist, always consult a medical professional for advice.

left: olive (*Olea europaea*)

colic

Colic may affect babies any time between birth and three or four months old. Severe abdominal pain, probably owing to gas in the immature digestive system, causes the baby to cry and to extend his or her legs or to pull them up toward the chest.

The Treatment Program

Many herbal remedies are unsuitable for babies, so the treatment plan below focuses on using homeopathy, which is perfectly safe from birth.

RECOMMENDED HOMEOPATHIC REMEDIES

Remedies can be given every half to one hour if the baby is in great discomfort. Use 6c or 30c potency. Dissolve one pill in a little cooled, boiled water and give the baby a teaspoon at a time. Make a fresh batch every 12 hours.

CHAMOMILLA, COLOCYNTHUS, DIOSCOREA, MAG PHOS This combination helps to relieve the cramping associated with colic, thus calming the baby.

tea for tinies

Fennel tea can be a great soother for a colicky baby. One of the main ingredients in fennel is a compound called anethole, which is found in fennel's essential oil. It is thought that anethole is chiefly responsible for reducing spasms in smooth muscle (such as that in the gastrointestinal tract) and therefore helps to relieve cramping. Serve as a weak, cold tea for babies. Steep one tea bag or 1 tsp of the herb in a cup of hot, once-boiled water for two minutes, strain if necessary, and then allow to cool. Give your baby 1 or 2 tsp of the tea immediately before and after each feed. You can keep a made-up batch of tea for up to 24 hours, then discard and make a fresh brew.

right: fennel (*Foeniculum vulgare*)

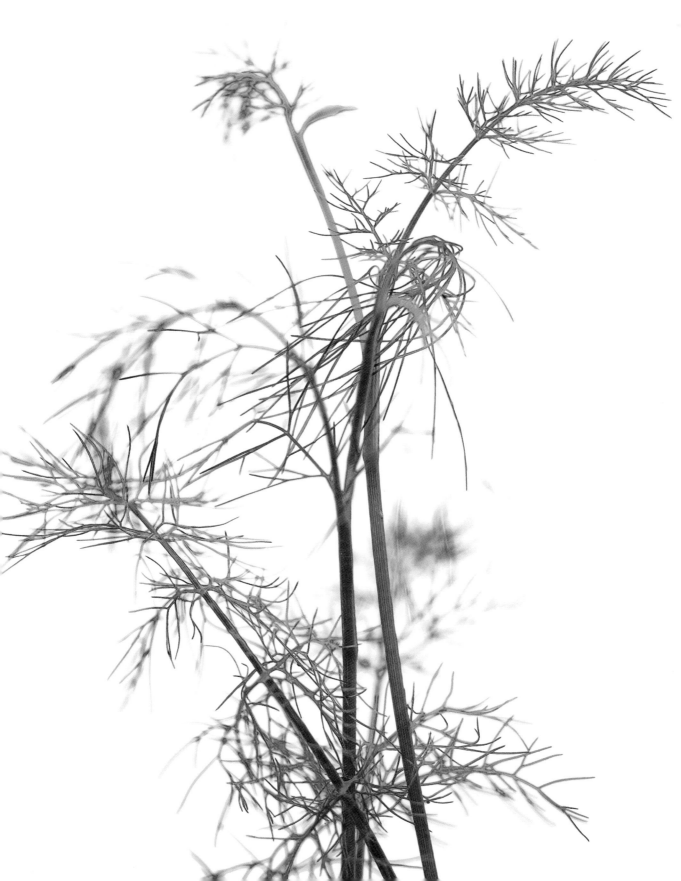

teething

A baby's first tooth may be an exciting time for parents, but for some babies teething can be very painful. The first tooth, usually a lower incisor, comes through at around the six-month stage (although it can be as early as three months or as late as 12 months). The pressure of teeth "cutting" through the gum, especially the blunt, double-edged molars at the back of the mouth, causes trauma and pain, often accompanied by flushed cheeks, sore gums, dribbling, irritability, mild fever (around 39°C/102°F), diarrhea, colic, loss of appetite and a desire to bite and chew.

The Treatment Program

Herbal remedies are not generally recommended for babies, but homeopathy and other simple techniques can be hugely effective at both reducing the pain and discomfort of teething and encouraging the teeth to come through quickly.

RECOMMENDED HOMEOPATHIC REMEDIES

Homeopathy works quickly and efficiently without any side effects. You can easily combine remedies and give them every half an hour if the baby is in great discomfort, in 6c or 30c potency. You can put two pillules directly into the mouths of babies who are older than three months; or you can crush or dissolve two pillules in a small amount of once-boiled, cooled water and give the remedy to your baby a teaspoon at a time.

CALCAREA CARBONICA If your baby's first teeth have not come through yet, "calc carb" can often kickstart the process; and if they have started to come through but are slow and causing discomfort, this remedy will help speed up the process. Calcarea carbonica is often suited to infants who are happy and plump.

CALCAREA PHOS AND CHAMOMILLA This combination is excellent for when your baby's gums are sore and inflamed, or if he or she is irritable and angry and will not be soothed. It is the best remedy to use when the baby's stools are loose and slightly green in colour, and the baby's face is flushed on one cheek.

BELLADONNA AND ACONITE This remedy is particularly useful when the baby's teething is accompanied by signs that the gums might be throbbing and extremely painful, and when the baby is restless. Also, it makes a good choice when the baby's face is hot and he or she has a slight fever.

PULSATILLA This remedy is wonderful for a baby who is very tearful during teething and becomes clingy and wants to be carried all the time. There may or may not be a green mucus discharge from the nose or in coughing, and generally the baby appears to feel worse in a warm room.

soothing the gums

There are many old wives' tales about how to ease the pain of teething – I'm sure that your mother and grandmother would have all sorts of advice for you, including perhaps rubbing alcohol into the gums, although we definitely don't recommend that now! However, there are a few traditional approaches that are worth preserving. The following are simple and often highly effective at soothing a teething baby's gums.

Carrot sticks If your baby is over six months old, giving him or her chilled carrot sticks to chew on will not only help with the pain, but will help teeth cut through the gum more easily. Be vigilant to make sure your baby doesn't choke, and once he or she as reached the age of one, if all the front teeth are through, abort the carrot sticks in favour of cold yogurt (see below) – a baby with his or her front teeth could bite off a chunk of carrot and choke on it. Never leave infants and small children alone while they are chewing on carrot sticks.

Yogurt Cold, but not frozen, yogurt can help to soothe gum pain. Give this remedy only to weaned children.

Water Boil a kettle, allow the water to cool, and then refrigerate it in a sterile container for 24 hours before giving it to your baby. The cold water will calm sore gums and is suitable for babies of all ages.

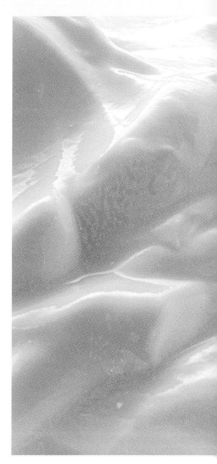

chicken pox

This highly contagious disease, which is most common in childhood but can occur at any time of life, is caused by the varicella zoster virus, a kind of herpes. One attack of chicken pox usually gives life-long immunity, although the virus can reactivate as shingles. After initial exposure, the virus incubates for between 14 and 21 days, after which spots begin to appear. The child is contagious until the spots crust over.

The Treatment Program

The first signs of chicken pox may be mistaken for a cold – headache, mild fever, sore throat and general malaise. Soon, however, an itchy, red rash develops, the spots of

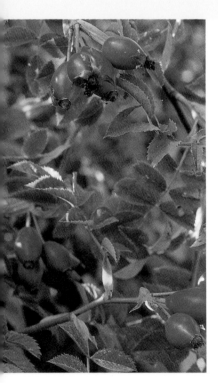

topical treatment to soothe the spots

Combine these topical creams with your internal treatment program for treating the illness. If you can't buy the calendula mixture ready-made, a good pharmacist or herbalist should be able to make it up for you using equal measures of each ingredient. You can use these creams on children at any age. Apply as often as you need to as relevant, unless otherwise directed.

Calendula, St John's wort, propolis cream Antiviral, antibacterial and soothing, these herbs will help to reduce irritation and inflammation and help the spots to heal more quickly.

Aloe vera gel Calming and soothing, a good-quality aloe vera gel will help to reduce inflammation and act as an antibacterial (preventing secondary infection). It is also very healing and will help to reduce itching.

Rose-hip seed oil Once the spots have crusted over, apply this oil undiluted twice a day to help prevent scarring.

which turn into fluid-filled vesicles, which usually last for between seven and ten days before drying up. The following program will help to fight the virus and ease symptoms.

RECOMMENDED HERBS

For children over two only, I recommend the following antiviral tonics. Give your child five drops of each tincture in a glass of water three times a day.

OLIVE LEAF (*Olea europaea*) Olive leaf contains the antiviral constituent oleuropein, which inhibits the activity of the herpes virus and may even help to destroy it.
ST JOHN'S WORT (*Hypericum perforatum*) Hypericin, hyperforin and flavonoids in St John's wort exhibit antiviral effects, and hypericin and hyperforin also support the nervous system, making St John's wort particularly useful against the herpes virus.

RECOMMENDED HOMEOPATHIC REMEDIES

As the symptoms of chicken pox can change every three to four days, it's important to change your remedy accordingly. For babies or younger children, dissolve one pill in a little once-boiled, cooled water and give one teaspoon every two or three hours. For older children give two pillules of 30c potency, three times a day.

ACONITE, BELLADONNA, FERRUM PHOS Use this in the early stages of chicken pox, when symptoms are cold-like, but you know your child has been exposed to the virus.
RHUS TOX, APIS, MEZEREUM This remedy treats the stage when the rash erupts.
PULSATILLA Use this remedy if your child is very weepy and clingy.
ANT TART OR ANT CRUD If the vesicles are accompanied by a cough or bronchitis, this remedy helps to ease the irritation in the lungs.
SULPHUR Toward the final days of the disease, sulphur helps to speed recovery.

NUTRITIONAL ADVICE

In weaned children the immune-boosting and anti-inflammatory foods recommended for coughs on page 79 (and viral infections; see p.61) help the body to fight chicken pox, too. Most importantly always make sure your child keeps up his or her fluid intake.

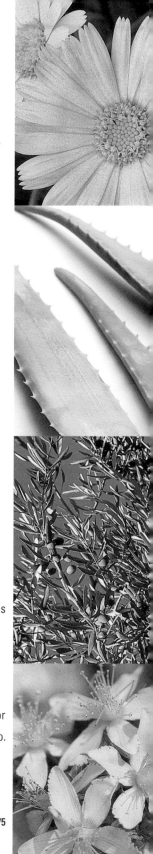

head lice

Head lice are small parasitic insects that live on the hair and scalp, and feed on the blood. Infestation is common among children – school children in particular. As head lice are unable to jump or fly, they rely upon physical head to head contact in order to spread. Contrary to popular belief, head lice do not target dirty hair; all hair is fair game. Lice are commonly referred to as nits. However, nits are the tiny, white eggs laid by the female lice and are not contagious. They attach firmly to the hair, near the root, and hatch in seven to ten days. It takes the baby lice (nymphs) a further seven to ten days to reach maturity, and adult lice can live for up to thirty days on the host, with each female louse laying up to one hundred eggs in that time.

The Treatment Program

Check your child regularly for nits or lice, especially if he or she is school-age or attends a nursery or pre-school. Signs that your child may have head lice include itching and scratching (although not everyone will experience these symptoms). However, the best way to tell is to use a louse or nit comb regularly. Nits will appear on the comb as tiny white flecks, rather like dandruff. My treatment program focuses on topical application and does not involve internal treatment at all.

RECOMMENDED TREATMENT

Conventional, commercial head-lice lotions and shampoos use pesticides that are not only toxic, but can be ineffective – over the years head lice have become resistant to some of them. However, nature has provided a wonderful, highly effective alternative.

NEEM (*Azadirachta indica*) This fantastic insecticide repels both lice and nits. Unlike its chemical counterparts, neem is not only effective, but lice do not seem to become resistant to it. It has no side effects and is suitable for children of all ages (and adults). It disrupts the lice's growth, feeding and reproduction cycles. Comb it through the infected hair once a day, without washing, for seven days. Treat the whole family.

making your own head lice oil

To 30ml/2 tbsp olive oil, add:

¾ tsp tea tree essential oil

10 drops rosemary essential oil

10 drops lavender essential oil

10 drops juniper essential oil

¼ tsp neem (this is usually sold as a solid, so you will need to put it in a little hot water to liquefy)

This mixture is suitable only for children over the age of two (see below for advice on treating very young children). Combine all the ingredients, or use The Organic Pharmacy's Neem Repellent Oil, and then pour the mixture, little by little, onto the child's head until you have covered the whole scalp. Using a fine-toothed, louse or nit comb (available from pharmacies), comb the oil mixture through the hair from root to tip all over the head. Be meticulous – take the hair in small sections and comb all the way down each time. The oil alone will make it difficult for the lice to move and the essential oils will have a therapeutic effect by killing both the eggs and the lice.

Once you have finished combing, leave the mixture on the hair for two to three hours or even overnight, and then shampoo it out. Because eggs hatch every seven days, you should repeat the combing process every two or three days for four cycles of seven days to make sure you have eradicated all the hatched eggs. Wash the comb in hot, soapy water between sessions.

For very young children

For children under the age of two, use only the olive oil and no essential oils. The oil will still make it hard for the lice to move and eventually eradicate them.

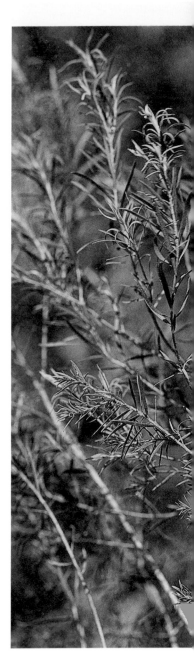

verrucae and warts

Verrucae and warts are caused by benign strains of the human papilloma virus (HPV). Warts are most commonly found on the hands (usually around the knuckles), while verrucae mainly grow on the soles of the feet and between the toes. Both are mildly contagious: warts can be passed through skin contact after the infected person has been scratching or picking at the wart, while a child is more likely to catch a verruca if his or her skin is wet and in contact with rough surfaces where infected people have been walking barefoot (such as around swimming pools). Children (or adults) with scratches or cuts on the soles of their feet are especially vulnerable to contracting the virus.

The Treatment Program

Effective childhood treatment of warts and verrucae involves building up the immature immune system using antiviral herbs, and treating with homeopathic remedies that address any underlying susceptibility to HPV. I have had great success with the following combination of treatments – in some cases, the verrucae or warts have disappeared within two weeks.

RECOMMENDED HERBS

I have suggested one herb for your child to take internally and one topical treatment. Using both approaches should give good results within four months. Both treatments are suitable for children of any age.

INTERNAL TREATMENT

For internal use, give your child 5 drops of the following herbal tincture diluted in a small amount of water twice a day for eight weeks.

OLIVE LEAF (*Olea europaea*) The main active constituent in olive leaf is a compound called oleuropein – and it is this that gives olive leaf its potent antiviral properties.

Oleuropein is thought to act by destroying the cell walls of a virus and by inhibiting the body's production of certain enzymes and amino acids, which the virus needs to grow and harm healthy cells. Olive leaf is also a good immune-booster.

TOPICAL TREATMENT

For the topical treatment, combine the tinctures of the following two herbs in equal measures, apply the mixture directly to the wart or verruca, allow it to dry and then place a band aid over the top to prevent the spread of infection. Repeat the application twice a day until the wart or verruca has gone. Never let your child take these herbs internally (and never take them internally yourself), owing to their powerful effects.

THUJA (*Thuja occidentalis*) Thuja has been used medicinally for centuries in Native North American cultures for its immune-boosting properties and potent antibacterial and antiviral effects.

CHELIDONIUM (*Chelidonium majus*) Also known as greater celandine, chelidonium has antimicrobial properties known to inhibit the human papilloma virus.

RECOMMENDED HOMEOPATHIC REMEDIES

Give your child the following homeopathic combination (which is suitable for children of all ages) in a 6c potency, twice a day until the wart or verruca has gone.

THUJA, ANT CRUD, CAUSTICUM, NIT AC This combination is excellent at attacking both warts and verrucae. It will also help to prevent their return.

NUTRITIONAL ADVICE

As warts and verrucae are caused by a virus, your child will need to eat plenty of immune-boosting foods, including lots of fresh fruit and vegetables, as well as garlic, ginger and cinnamon (see also the nutritional advice for bacterial and viral infections on page 61). It is more important than ever to steer you child well clear of junk foods – these will only deplete an already strained immune system, making the recovery and healing time that much longer.

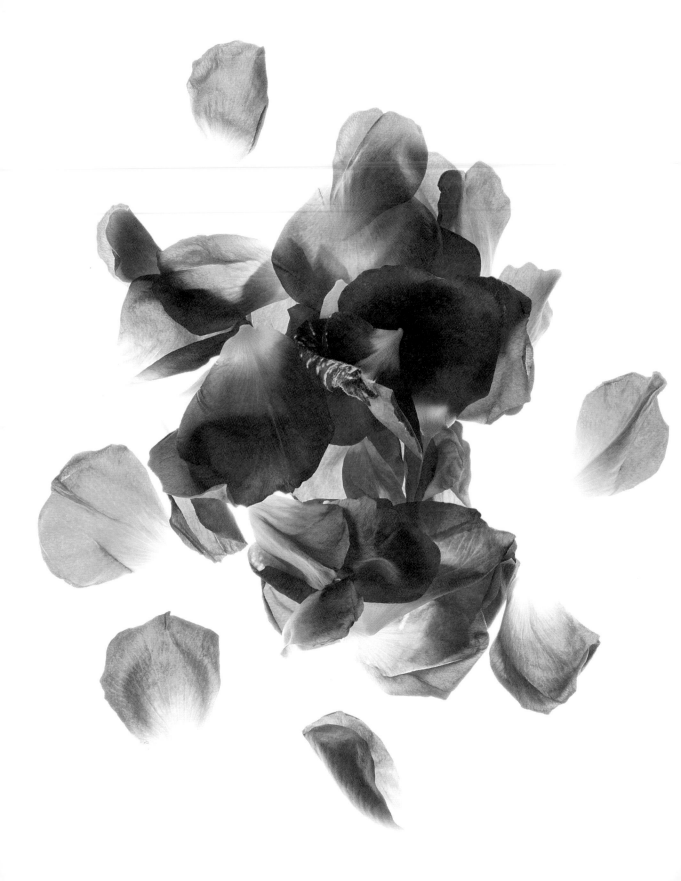

CHAPTER 8

ultimate skin care

People often think of their skin merely as a shell, the part of them that's on the outside to keep all the other bits inside and together. However, the skin – and specifically its appearance – is much more than a shell: it is a wonderful barometer of your health. This means ultimate skin care has to begin with what you put into your body – the food you eat, the fluids you drink, the air you breathe, and the cosmetics you use. In addition, your skin needs tender, loving care of its own, with an established routine that uses pure ingredients. Looking after your skin, and your well-being, is not about vanity – it's a sign that you care about yourself and your health.

Just as I am a fervent believer in eating fresh, organic produce, I believe that what you put onto your skin should be as natural as possible, without any of the added chemicals and artificial fragrances that go in to many of today's cosmetics. These "regular" cosmetics simply add to your toxic load and impair your general health. Organic is always best – whether it's on the inside or the outside of your body. Over the following pages I am absolutely thrilled to be able to give you my personal organic skin-care regime. It isn't a quick-fix, and at times it may seem hard to follow, but by committing to the care of your skin using my approaches, I promise you youthfulness, beauty and good skin health for years to come.

left: rose petals (*Rosa damascena*)

understanding your skin

Your skin is a living, breathing organ – the largest in the body. As well as affecting the way you look and feel, the skin has several crucial functions. First, it forms a physical barrier against invading microbes. Second, it allows you to touch and feel. And third, it helps to maintain your body temperature, stores and synthesizes vitamin D, provides a system of elimination by allowing you to expel toxins through sweat and absorbs oxygen and other nutrients. In short, your skin is very busy! Billions of cells work together to perform all these vital functions throughout the skin's three layers: the epidermis, dermis and subcutaneous layer.

THE LAYERS OF THE SKIN

THE EPIDERMIS The uppermost layer of the skin, the epidermis is made up of stacked layers of cells that overlap each other, like tiles on a roof, and are glued together by protein bridges known as desmosomes. The lowest layer of the epidermis itself is called the basal layer (see diagram, opposite). It is from the basal layer that all the cells of the epidermis originate. Their function is to replace the dead cells that slough off from the top of the skin. As they move upward, the living epidermal cells produce keratin,

water – your beauty secret

Water makes up thirty percent of the epidermis, the skin's outermost layer (see diagram, opposite). If you want fresh-looking skin, then water is essential. The process of water moving through the body to the surface of the skin is called "transepidermal water loss". If you are dehydrated, the body holds back water, preventing transepidermal water loss from taking place, so that the skin's upper layers become dry and brittle. Fixing this couldn't be easier: all you have to do is to drink at least six glasses of water every day and eat lots of fresh fruits and vegetables, which are all water-rich.

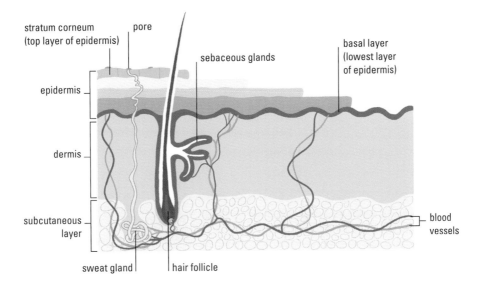

stratum corneum
(top layer of epidermis)

pore

sebaceous glands

basal layer
(lowest layer
of epidermis)

epidermis

dermis

subcutaneous
layer

blood
vessels

sweat gland

hair follicle

a protein that protects the skin. Gradually, as they journey through the layers of the epidermis, these cells lose their nuclei and become thin, flat and hexagonal-shaped – at which point they die. Even as they die, they are bound together so that the skin creates a waterproof barrier. Eventually these dead cells slough off, too, only to be replaced with fresh cells from the basal layer. The whole process takes between twenty and 28 days, depending upon your age (the older you are, the longer it takes).

THE SKIN'S NATURAL MOISTURIZER

The uppermost layer of the epidermis is called the stratum corneum. This layer contains a number of water-soluble chemicals – including amino acids, lactic acid and urea – that form the skin's Natural Moisturizing Factor (NMF). NMF protects the skin by retaining water to keep the stratum corneum hydrated. In addition, the cells of the stratum corneum are surrounded by certain fats called intercellular lipids (which include cholesterol, ceramides and fatty acids), the job of which is to "trap" NMF and water in the skin and prevent their loss through perspiration. There are sharp decreases in the numbers of intercellular lipids in the stratum corneum after the age of forty, which

caring for oily skin

Oily skin produces excessive amounts of sebum. It is tempting to remove this oil by using oil-free products. However, this only makes the skin dry up, prompting the sebaceous glands to produce even more oil. The result is usually combination skin, with dry and oily patches, as well as enlarged pores. If you have oily skin, I recommend you stay away from oil-free products. Use "light" cosmetics that contain small amounts of oil to balance the skin naturally.

makes people over forty more susceptible to dry-skin conditions. Solvents, detergents, soap and other chemicals can damage the stratum corneum, stripping away the lipids and leading to the loss of NMF. This is why it is so important to avoid using cosmetic and soap products that contain harsh detergents.

THE DERMIS Beneath the epidermis lies the dermis. This thick layer of fibrous and elastic tissue is made up of eighty percent collagen and twenty percent elastin. These proteins give the skin its strength and elasticity, respectively. The dermis also contains blood vessels that serve the basal layer of the epidermis (see pp.182–183). Also in the dermis are sebaceous glands, which secrete sebum, an oil-like substance that protects the hair and skin; and lymph vessels, which drain away waste products from the skin and destroy micro-organisms in the skin as part of the immune response. In addition, the dermis contains nerve endings, sweat glands and hair follicles. The principle type of cell in the dermis is the fibroblast, which synthesizes collagen, elastin and other structural molecules.

THE SUBCUTANEOUS LAYER The deepest layer of the skin is the subcutaneous layer. A layer of connective tissue and fat cells, it supports the blood vessels that feed essential nutrients to the other layers of the skin, provides cushioning against bumps, offers a layer of insulation to keep the body warm, and helps to keep the other layers of the skin in place.

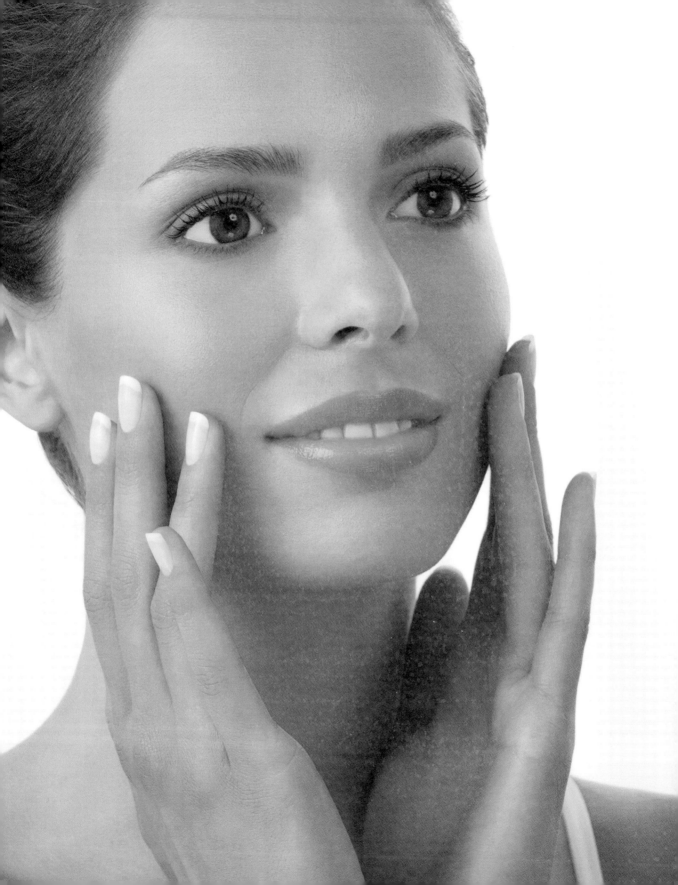

caring for your skin: on the outside

Good topical skin care means establishing a thorough skin-care routine that uses the right products. Many skin-care preparations use artificial preservatives, colourants and fragrances, as well as chemicals that strip your skin of its moisture and natural oils. I want you to know which ingredients you should look out for – to buy and to avoid – so that you are fully armed to have a skin-care clear-out that will then enable you to have skin-care make-over, beginning with my routine on the opposite page.

BUYING ORGANIC

Your skin will absorb whatever you put onto it. This means that if your cosmetics contain toxins, your skin may well absorb some of them. For example, some research has shown that harmful ingredients such as parabens are able to penetrate the skin to be released into the blood stream. Choosing cosmetics carefully is vital. In organic skin-care products, the herbs and other plant ingredients have been grown without the use of pesticides, artificial fertilizers and so on – just as with organic foods. This means that organic cosmetics do not contain some of the known carcinogens and other harmful chemicals that are in many standard cosmetic products. Research has also shown that organic extracts contain higher levels of nutrients than non-organic products to keep your skin well-nourished, and so healthy and beautiful-looking.

INGREDIENTS TO AVOID

Avoid any cosmetics that contain the following, harmful chemicals:
• parabens (parahydroxy benoic acid) • artificial fragrances • detergents (sodium lauryl sulphate and sodium laureth sulphate) • nitrosamine precursors (these are DEA and TEA, which react with nitrites to become carcinogenic nitrosamines) • formaldehyde-releasing preservatives (quarternium 15, imidazolidinyl urea, DMDM hydrantoin, 2-bromo-2-nitropropane-1, 3-diol) • propylene glycerol • phthalates

your daily skin-care routine

The following is my personal recommendation for a daily skin-care routine. All the usual stages are here – cleansing, toning and moisturizing – with my personal advice on what to use and when to use it for blemish-free, beautiful skin.

CLEANSING

It is crucial to cleanse. Dirt, pollution, grime and make-up mix with the skin's natural moisturizer sebum and, if not removed with a cleanser, can clog up the pores to dull the skin and even cause spots.

WHAT TO USE As sebum is oily, the best cleanser is one that is oil-based, which you then remove with a face cloth that has been soaked in hand hot water and wrung out. Oily skin will benefit from this, too, because the procedure helps remove excess sebum (see box, p.134).

WHEN TO CLEANSE The most important time to cleanse is at night, when I prefer to use a balm (an oil-based cleanser). In the morning, I use a gentle face wash or milk. Cleansing more than twice a day is unnecessary and may irritate the skin.

protecting the skin's mantle

When sebum (the skin's natural oil) and sweat mix on the surface of the skin they form a protective barrier known as the acid mantle. This makes the skin less vulnerable to damage by factors such as the sun and wind, and less likely to dry out. It also inhibits the growth of foreign bacteria and fungi in the skin, keeping it blemish-free. Regular soap can strip away the acid mantle, making your skin vulnerable. To help prevent this, avoid using ordinary soaps, and instead opt for balm (oil-based) cleansers, cleansing milks, and gels that are free from harsh detergents.

TONING

Most toners remove the residues of a cleanser. However, think of your toner as your primary moisturizer, giving water and nutrients back to your skin.

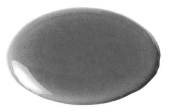

WHAT TO USE Use a toner packed with herbal extracts that repair the skin. Aloe vera and rose are great for all skin types; rose on its own is excellent for dry skin. Use a combination of aloe with a herb such as lavender or calendula for oily skin; and with lemon or gotu kola for combination skin.

WHEN TO TONE You should tone your skin twice a day, morning and night.

MOISTURIZING

A moisturizer protects the skin from the elements and increases the water content of the stratum corneum (see pp.183–184). One way moisturizers do this is by having ingredients that restore the lipid barrier of the skin's cells – beeswax, plant oils and a mineral oil known as petrolatum are such ingredients. (Note: petrolatum can hinder other functions in the skin, such as allowing it to "breathe".) Other ingredients in moisturizers, called humecants and including glycerin and sorbitol, rehydrate the skin.

WHAT TO USE You need two kinds of moisturizer. The first is a full-scale, cream-based moisturizer that includes lipid restorers and humecants. All the "star" ingredients in this book make miraculous components for full moisturizing creams. Take a list of them everywhere, so that you can always check a product's label before you buy. The second kind of moisturizer is a face oil or, for those with very oily skin, a gel that contains small amounts of oil. Remember that quality is essential. Look for oils that are cold-pressed, organic and rich in colour – these are all signs of a good oil.

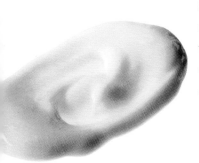

WHEN TO MOISTURIZE You should moisturize twice a day. Use your full moisturizing cream in the morning and the face oil or gel at night.

the three-minute DIY facial

The younger we are, the quicker the renewal of cells in the epidermis (see pp.182–183), which is what keeps us looking young. A facial every 28 days greatly enhances this cycle of skin-cell regeneration, while gentle massage on the face improves blood-flow to the skin and stimulates the movement of lymph (see p.29), which, unlike the blood, has no pumping action of its own.

However, even without a salon facial every month, giving yourself this simple, three-minute, at-home facial massage as part of your daily cleansing routine, helps to recontour your face, reduce puffiness and give your complexion that all-important glow.

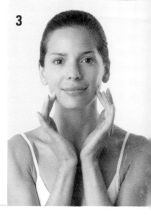

1 With a little cleanser or treatment serum applied to your fingers and palms, beginning at the centre of your brow, swipe outward moving your hands away from one another toward your ears and then down your neck. Repeat this motion, this time beginning beneath your eyes (fingers either side of your nose), then out toward your ears and down the sides of your neck; and then again, this time beginning beneath your nose at the middle of your top lip.

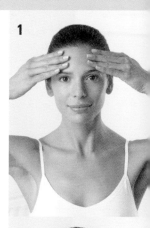

2 Apply more cleanser or treatment serum as necessary, then using the fingers of both hands, begin at your chin and swipe outward toward your ears and down the sides of your neck.

3 Beginning at your temples, swipe down the sides of your face and down your neck. Then finish by gently sweeping your fingers up your neck and across your cheeks, using superficial tapping movements.

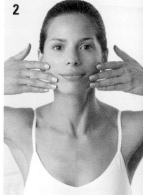

caring for your skin:
on the inside

Although dry or oily skin can be a result of poor topical skin care, they can also be a result of poor internal health. Dry skin may indicate a lack of sebum to nourish the skin's upper cells, not enough protein to bind cells or general dehydration in the body. Both dry and oily skin can result from hormonal imbalance. A detox will greatly enhance the body's ability to restore balance to the upper layers of the skin through better oxygenation and elimination. Supplying your skin with the right nutrients will also enhance its appearance, helping to make it clear and fresh.

DETOXIFYING YOUR SKIN

Cleansing is the single most important step in the external care of your skin – and it is the single most important internal step, too. When the body accumulates toxins, the main organs of elimination (see pp.28–29) aim to get rid of them as quickly as possible. However, an excessive build-up of toxins can overload these organs, making the skin the natural outlet for the excess. As waste accumulates in the skin's layers, it is more difficult for oxygen and nutrients to access cells, and the skin becomes starved, dull, lifeless, puffy and spotty. With prolonged toxic overload, the skin loses its ability to regenerate its cells, resulting in a loss of firmness. So, if you want beautiful skin, the first step you must take is the ten-day detox on pages 50–53. Whether you are boosting the appearance of tired-looking skin or trying to overcome the effects of eczema, acne, dermatitis, pigmentation (liver spots) or aging, a detox will almost always show results.

FEEDING YOUR SKIN

The skin needs a ready supply of nutrients. After water and oxygen, antioxidants and lipids are the most important skin nutrients as they are essential for skin-renewal. In addition, other essential nutrients, such as essential fatty acids and vitamin B, will help to keep your skin supple, help it to do its work as an organ and encourage the skin cells to multiply and regenerate. Try to increase all of the following in your diet.

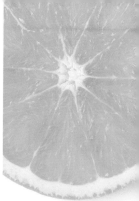

OLIGOMERIC PROANTHOCYANIDINS (OPCs) OPCs protect cells, support immunity and moderate inflammation (which occurs in nearly all skin conditions).

FIND THEM IN Bilberries • cranberries • grapes • green tea • pine bark extract

ALPHA LIPOIC ACID (ALA) The antioxidant ALA also boosts the action of vitamins C and E (see below) and stimulates the liver to produce the protein antioxidant glutathione. You will need to take ALA in supplement form because, although spinach, broccoli, organ meats, Brewer's yeast and beef all contain ALA, food sources have little effect on blood levels, making supplementation necessary.

VITAMIN A AND OTHER CAROTENOIDS These increase the rate of cell division in your skin, promoting renewal.

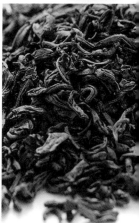

FIND THEM IN Brightly coloured fruits and vegetables (including carrots, red peppers, sweet potatoes, Cantaloupe melon and mangoes) • eggs • kale • spinach

SELENIUM This mineral protects the skin tissues and is a component in the enzyme glutathione peroxidase, which protects organs from oxidative damage.

FIND IT IN Eggs • grains • legumes • nuts (particularly Brazil nuts) • oats • tuna

VITAMIN (ESTER) C One of the most powerful and effective antioxidants, vitamin C also has a major role to play in the formation of collagen, which keeps the skin elastic.

FIND IT IN Broccoli • cabbage • citrus fruits • kiwis • red peppers

VITAMIN E This fat-soluble vitamin protects the lipid layer from oxidation.

FIND IT IN Avocados • cereals (especially wheat) • herring • nuts (particularly hazelnuts, Brazil nuts, and peanuts) • pine nuts

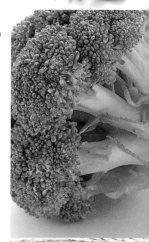

ZINC This essential mineral can help to regulate the oil production of cells, as well as promote tissue repair. Your skin needs it for protein synthesis and collagen formation.

FIND IT IN Eggs • lentils • peas • red meat • shellfish • spinach

OTHER BEAUTY NUTRIENTS

ESSENTIAL FATTY ACIDS (EFAs) The building blocks of the lipids that protect the skin's cells (see p.183), EFAs enable cells to repair and regenerate.

FIND THEM IN Oily fish (such as tuna and salmon) • pumpkin seeds • sunflower seeds • walnuts. (Note: For your body to absorb and utilize EFAs properly it needs a good

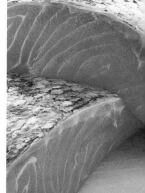

supply of EFA co-factors. These include substances such as choline, biotin and lecithin, which can be found in nuts, eggs, green leafy vegetables and soy products.)

B-COMPLEX VITAMINS The B-vitamins are essential for your body's metabolism of proteins and fats (which are essential for skin health), and for the skin's protection against the harmful rays of the sun.

FIND THEM IN Asparagus • green leafy vegetables • eggs • milk • watercress

METHYLSULFONYLAMINE (MSM) A sulphur-like complex found in both plants and animals, MSM helps to detoxify the body, reduce inflammation and nourish the skin.

FIND IT IN Cucumber • fennel • garlic • onion • radish • raw fresh fruits and vegetables

superfoods for beautiful skin

There are some foods that your skin just cries out for you to eat, because they are so densely packed with the vitamins and minerals that it needs to stay healthy and so look beautiful. The following are my skin superfoods – I urge you to eat them whenever you can.

Alfalfa Packed with calcium, magnesium, potassium, chlorophyll, betacarotene, B-vitamins and more, alfalfa is a great all-in-one source of antioxidants and green foods (see below). Calcium and magnesium are essential for tissue repair.

Green foods – barley grass, wheatgrass, spirulina and chlorella These foods are a combination of micro algae and sprouted grains. All are rich in chlorophyll, which has a unique ability to cleanse the cells of toxins such as heavy metals (including mercury and lead) and pesticides, as well as being packed full with vitamins C, E and betacarotene, and minerals, amino acids and essential fatty acids.

Goji berries The Chinese goji berry (sometimes called the wolf berry) is packed with nutrients – including carotenoids and vitamins C, B1, B2 and B3; as well as 18 amino acids, which are the building blocks for proteins such as collagen and elastin, and minerals, such as zinc, selenium, calcium and iron. This skin superfood rejuvenates and regenerates your skin's cells.

right: wheatgrass (*Triticum aestivum*)

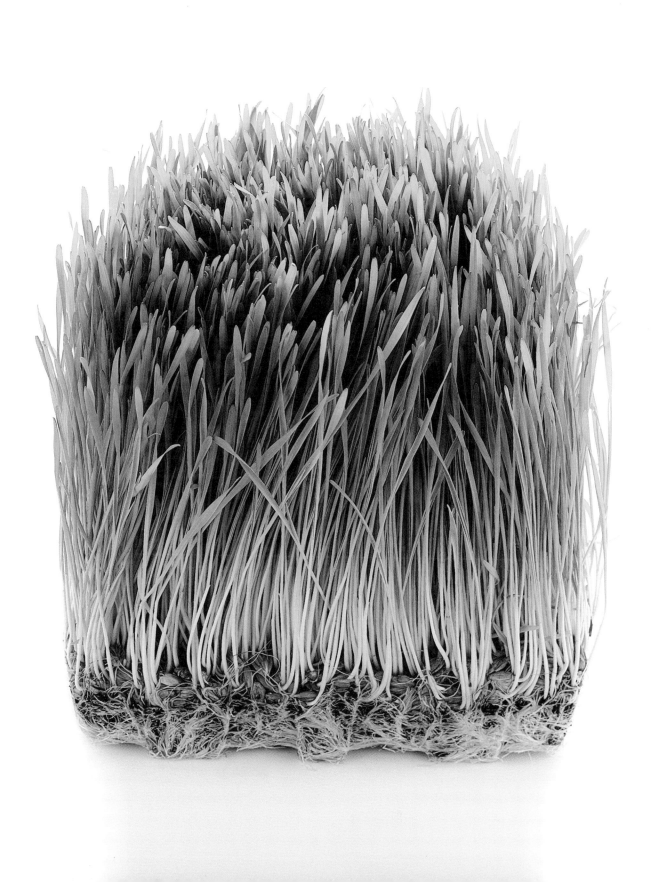

anti-aging: skin care
to stay young

Looking younger for longer is really relatively simple: the dermis, the second layer of your skin (beneath the epidermis, the uppermost layer), has a high content of collagen and elastin fibres, which keep the skin strong and supple. All you need to do to maintain your skin's youthful appearance is to keep the dermis healthy.

THE SKIN'S PROTEINS

Collagen, which forms the structural network of skin, is the most abundant protein in the body and one of the strongest in nature – it is what gives your skin its strength. However, as you age, or if collagen becomes damaged (for example, through over-exposure to the UV rays in sunlight), this protein can become cross-linked, which means that the collagen fibres lose their flexibility and become rigid, resulting in dull, wrinkled, sagging skin. Elastin, also a protein, is more "stretchable" than collagen and maintains the skin's elasticity. Like collagen, it breaks down as you age, causing wrinkles.

HOW DO WE DAMAGE OUR SKIN?

No one can prevent aging. However, all sorts of environmental factors increase the load on your skin, making the aging process more apparent. If you can identify these factors, and minimize them, you can slow down the rate at which you appear to age.

Harsh skin-care regimes destroy the acid mantle of the skin (see p.187); toxins in many commercial skin-care products, and in the environment, can all contribute to cross-linking in your collagen fibres; and the UV rays in sunlight, as well as cigarette smoke, a poor diet, too much alcohol, dehydration, stress and lack of sleep, are lifestyle contributors to skin damage. Many of these factors have one common link – the free radical. Essentially, skin damage (and what we see as skin-aging) occurs when the membrane of a skin cell is damaged by free radicals. This makes the membrane more permeable, allowing the cells to dehydrate. Just as the stratum corneum needs its protective lipid layer (see p.183), so skin cells need their protective membrane.

WHAT ARE FREE RADICALS AND WHAT CAN WE DO ABOUT THEM?

Free radicals are unstable atoms that are generated as the body consumes oxygen to create energy. They occur in every cell throughout your body simply by virtue of the fact that oxygen is your principal metabolic fuel, and they can damage and destroy cell membranes and even a cell nucleus. Your body's metabolism is the process the body goes through to break down your food to find nutrition and expel waste. Some free radicals are simply its natural by-product.

In addition, the UV rays in sunlight generate free radicals in the skin, as does exposure to other environmental toxins, including cigarette smoke and radiation. Free radicals are also produced when you consume certain heated cooking oils (including sunflower and rapeseed oils) and hydrogenated fats. When you are stressed, your body makes more free radicals than normal. Stress also causes the body to use up nutrients more quickly, which means they don't reach your skin to nourish and hydrate it. Some of these nutrients are antioxidants, and these provide the key to minimizing the effects of free radicals in the body, because they "mop up" the unstable atoms. Take a look at the lists on page 191 and see how to boost antioxidant-rich foods in your diet.

the ultimate inside and out smoothie

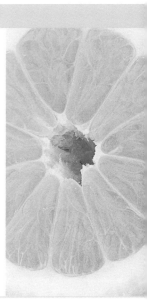

4 plums, pitted, flesh chopped
20 goji berries
juice of ½ a lemon
125ml/4fl oz/½ cup of water

I discovered the benefits of this drink on my skin by accident. I wanted to alkalize my body (high acidity destroys cells) and feed it some supernutrients, so I blended these ingredients. As my skin needed some tender loving care, once I'd sipped most of the smoothie, I scooped up some of the remains and applied them to my skin, leaving the mixture there for five minutes. I couldn't believe the results: my skin was instantly smooth, velvety and radiant! Whiz the ingredients in a blender, then try it inside – and out.

creating your anti-aging plan

Over the following pages I've revealed some of the best and most effective topical anti-aging agents I've come across – they include antioxidants (which studies show applied topically can reverse skin-aging), nutrients to reverse the natural slowing down of the skin's ability to repair and renew itself, and herbs that promote good micro-capillary action, which in turn feeds your skin with essential nutrients and oxygen, and carries waste products away. I've chosen my favourites, but there are simply hundreds of others I could have also included, which is part of what I love about my work. One of the most exciting aspects is researching and exploring new or even old extracts that I can use in different ways. It's time now for you to discover the topical anti-aging secrets of Nature's kingdom.

The Topical Treatment Program

The following anti-aging plan focuses on topical treatment, but this doesn't mean that what you put into your body won't affect the aging of your skin. Read the general

taking care of older skin

If you are 45 or older, it's more important than ever to look after your skin – and it's never too late to start and to make up good ground in the race to look younger. After the age of 45, as the balance of hormones changes in your body, your skin (whatever your sex) becomes thinner and more vulnerable to attack from free radicals and environmental pollution. Skin also tends to heal more slowly as a result of slower cell renewal. Take extra-special care to follow my daily skin-care routine (see pp.187–189), every day, and look for products that contain the heroes among nature's moisturizers, such as aloe (see pp.106–107), which is especially hydrating, and lovely rose (see pp.200–201), which helps to protect your skin.

skin-care advice on pages 187–189, too, and complement this with the following topical recommendations. Finally, your plan must limit your exposure to known free-radical triggers (see p.195) and include plenty of filtered or bottled water (to keep the cells hydrated) – drink at least six glasses a day (see box, p.182).

RECOMMENDED HERBS

The natural world is packed with herbs and nutrients that effectively accelerate and enhance the skin's processes of repair and regeneration. The following herbs, applied topically, are essential for an effective anti-aging regime. Look for creams, oils and serums containing these ingredients and apply them twice a day as part of your daily skin-care program.

PINE BARK EXTRACT (*Pinus maritima*) This herb protects the skin by binding to elastin and collagen and preventing their breakdown, so reducing wrinkles. The herb also protects the tiny capillaries in the skin and restores good blood circulation, assuring the supply of nutrients and oxygen to the skin, and removing waste.

KIGELIA (*Kigelia africana*) Studies have shown kigelia (also known by the delightful name "the African sausage tree") to be rich in derivatives of caffeic acid – a compound with strong antioxidant properties. Kigelia also has a potent anti-inflammatory action on the skin, helping it to repair itself, and contains hormone-like substances that are mainly responsible for firming the skin.

CALENDULA (*Calendula officinalis*) The king of the herbs when it comes to beating back the clock, calendula acts on aging skin in three main ways. First, at a time when blood supply to the skin is diminishing, calendula helps to create new blood vessels in the skin. Second, it's packed full of carotenoid pigments and lutein, the antioxidant effects of which fight free-radical damage. And finally, research shows that calendula actually stimulates collagen synthesis and cell regeneration for younger-looking skin. It is one of my star ingredients (see pp.126–127).

GOTU KOLA (*Centella asiatica*) Gotu kola has many different actions on the skin, each contributing to its extraordinary results. First, as an anti-inflammatory, this herb activates collagen synthesis and slows collagen breakdown. Its effect on the

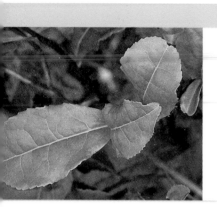

green tea

Green tea contains polyphenols (plant chemicals) that are twenty times stronger than the beneficial plant chemicals found in vitamin E. As a result, applied to the skin, green tea protects skin cells from damage by free radicals. In addition, xanthines (a group of alkaloids) in green tea act as a potent anti-inflammatory. Good natural pharmacies and skin-care boutiques will sell products that contain green tea.

micro-circulation helps to improve cell nutrition and detoxification. Finally, it rebalances the keratinization process (the replenishment of keratin in cells) of the stratum corneum (see p.183), so thwarting moisture-loss and restoring the skin's integrity.

ALOE VERA (*Aloe vera*) The active ingredients in aloe vera are so potent that this plant has clearly demonstrable healing, anti-inflammatory, cell renewal, and moisturizing effects on the skin. Always use aloe vera extract of the highest quality. Aloe is another of my star ingredients (see pp.106–107).

BILBERRY (*Vaccinium myrtillus*) When you eat bilberries, the antioxidant-rich fruit works internally to fight free radicals and improve micro-circulation – and they do exactly the same when applied externally, too!

RECOMMENDED NUTRIENTS

Although most of the following nutrients help to improve the quality of your skin if you take them internally (either through food or as supplements), I have chosen these specifically with topical treatment in mind. At The Organic Pharmacy we have formulated several topical treatments containing them, all without the use of toxins. Look out for the nutrients in all the beauty products that you buy.

VITAMIN (ESTER) C Recent research shows that applying vitamin C to the skin can reduce inflammation, wrinkle formation, and unwanted pigmentation such as liver spots.

It can also increase collagen formation, maintaining or even increasing the skin's suppleness. In particular, ester C (a fat-soluble, non-acidic form of vitamin C) is important because it protects both the fat and water portions of cells, helps to reduce any micro-inflammation that interferes with the skin's elasticity, and regenerates vitamin E in the skin, which we need to provide antioxidant protection in the skin's elastin fibres. However, always seek advice from your doctor, natural pharmacist, or dermatologist before applying vitamin-C cream. Ultimately, vitamin C is an acid (ascorbic acid) and high levels can damage the skin in exactly the same way as a chemical burn.

VITAMIN A AND OTHER CAROTENOIDS These nutrients are wonderful at repairing the signs of aging that result from sun exposure. Studies have shown they stimulate the growth of fibroplasts (cells that help with the formation of connective tissue), encourage collagen synthesis and prevent collagen breakdown. Topical treatments that contain rose-hip seed oil (see p.151) will be rich in vitamin A and carotenoids. (Rose-hip seed oil is also rich in essential fatty acids, which are vital as we get older to replenish moisture in the skin.)

ALPHA LIPOIC ACID Water-soluble and fat-soluble, alpha lipoic acid is able to protect both the water-based and fat-based portions of the skin's cells. Applied topically, this nutrient acts as not only as an antioxidant but also as a collagen-booster helping to reinstate firmness to the skin. It also boosts the actions of the antioxidant vitamins C and E in the body.

GLUCOSAMINE Although better known for its action on the joints, ligaments and muscles, glucosamine may be the hottest anti-aging ingredient of the moment. Recent research shows that, when applied topically to the skin, it is able to reduce the amount of melanin in skin cells and therefore unwanted pigmentation, such as liver spots. Tissue studies using glucosamine also show that this compound helps to increase collagen production.

Although I've listed my favourite anti-aging treatments here, scientists, pharmacists and herbalists are making new discoveries about the beneficial properties of plants all the time. Keep your eyes peeled for news of what's new in natural skin-care.

STAR INGREDIENT: rose

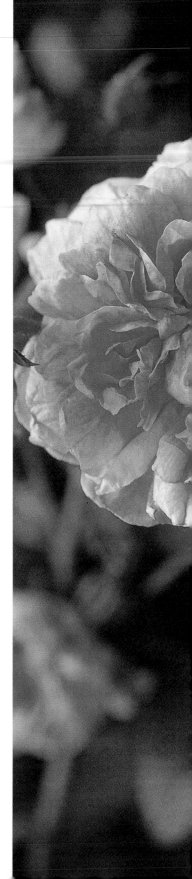

More than a decade ago, I was travelling through Kerman, Iran, when I came across a local rose harvest. An entire village had come together to pick rose petals at dawn, when the flowers' essential-oil content is at its greatest. Little stalls were set up along the tracks with tiny silver vials containing the oil. As I opened a vial and inhaled, the unique, heady smell of rose took my breath away. Two days later I came across a Bakhtiari tribe settlement. As I sat drinking delicious rose tea, I watched as the Bakhtiari women applied an oil to their faces. These women lead hard lives, mostly outdoors in the sun and wind, and it surprised me that their skin was so smooth and glowing. I asked them their secret and they readily shared it – rose oil mixed with sunflower oil.

Understanding Rose

Fresh leaves and flowers are steam-distilled to produce rose water and rose essential oil, although it is also possible to isolate the oil using solvent extraction (in this case the oil is called rose "absolute"). I recommend buying a steam-distilled rose oil as this yields a purer, and therefore more therapeutic, extract. It takes 40,000kg (45 tons) of rose petals to make 1kg (2 lb) of rose oil, making it more expensive than gold.

Rose (*Rosa damascena*) is a mixture of more than 300 compounds, some of which scientists have yet to identify. These compounds give rose countless therapeutic qualities – its most important actions on the body and mind are given in the lists below.

FOR THE SKIN

ANTI-AGING Roses contain plant pigments called anthocyanins. These are powerful antioxidants (see p.195) that protect the rose plant from "photo damage" by the harmful UV rays in sunlight. Amazingly, anthocyanins can also protect our skin cells when applied topically (as an oil) or taken internally (as a tea). They also strengthen the capillaries in the skin and inhibit the breakdown of elastin (see p.194), making rose a favourite for anti-aging treatments.

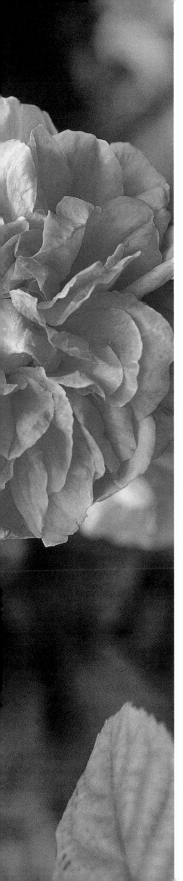

TO REDUCE REDNESS AND BROKEN CAPILLARIES Antioxidant and anti-inflammatory, vitamin B3 (nicotinamide) is a key ingredient in rose oil. This nutrient aids the circulation and helps to keep the skin free from broken veins and redness.

TO HEAL INFLAMMATION Rose contains the flavonoid quercetin, which studies have shown may inhibit the formation of pro-inflammatory prostaglandins – compounds that cause swelling. It also contains anti-inflammatory compounds called polyphenols and carotenoids. According to research, quercetin may also block the enzyme that breaks down elastin, helping to keep skin supple and smooth.

FOR HEALTH

TO INCREASE FERTILITY As it contains astringent tannins, which can harmonize menstrual flow, rose is a great choice for improving reproductive health in women. Rose also helps to cleanse the body and has been shown to increase the sperm count in men.

TO IMPROVE MOOD Rose essential oil is well known for its uplifting action on the mind. While there has been no firm research on this aspect of rose's activity, the oil's amazing mood-enhancing effect is thought to be a result of its action on the hypothalamus, a part of your brain that is linked to the limbic system, which in turn is involved with the control of your emotions.

the story of rose essential oil

The wonderful story of the Persian princess who married the Mughal King Shah Jahangir in India in the 1600s is perhaps the first story of the discovery of rose essential oil. The story goes that the king asked his builders to construct a large canal in the gardens of the palace and fill it with rose water. In the burning heat of the Indian sun, the oil and the water separated, creating a film of oil that floated on the water's surface. The princess was taken by its exquisite smell and asked that it be collected as a perfume, or *attar* (essential oil).

table of herbs

herb	actions/indications	contraindications
agnus castus (*Vitex agnus castus*)	PMS, acne, increased milk production	Avoid if you are also taking dopaminergic agonists or antagonists
aloe vera (*Aloe vera*)	Anti-aging; wounds, gastric problems	None known
anise (*Pimpinella anisum*)	Coughs, bloating, colic	None known
arnica (*Arnica montana*)	Bruising, swelling, muscular or rheumatic aches	Toxic internally as a herb (but fine in homeopathic form). Externally, apply only to unbroken skin
ashwaganda (*Withania somnifera*)	Anti-aging; exhaustion, convalescence, stress, poor memory	Avoid if taking sleeping pills or tranquillizers (or other sedatives), or after alcohol
astragalus (*Astragalus membranaceus*)	Cancer support; coughs, colds, fatigue, stress	Avoid if you are also taking immunosuppressive medication
bilberry (*Vaccinium myrtillus*)	Eye tonic; diarrhea, hemorrhoids, broken capillaries, poor circulation	None known in recommended doses. Long-term use can lead to constipation
black cohosh (*Cimicifuga racemosa*)	Arthritic and muscular pain, menopausal symptoms	None known
bogbean (*Menyanthes trifoliata*)	Arthritis, rheumatoid and muscular arthritis	None known in recommended doses. Excessive doses can cause diarrhea, nausea and vomiting
burdock (*Arctium lappa*)	Skin eruptions such as acne; rheumatism, cystitis	None known
calendula (*Calendula officinalis*)	Anti-aging; cuts, sores, infections, skin problems	None known
cardamom (*Elettaria cardamomum*)	Bad breath, sore throats, colic, bloating	None known
cat's claw (*Uncaria tomentosa*)	Infections, cancer, arthritis	If taking immunosuppressive drugs seek the advice of a practitioner. Avoid with anticoagulant drugs
chelidonium (*Chelidonium majus*)	Warts, verrucae, liver protector, promotion of bile	Avoid if pregnant
chickweed (*Stellaria media*)	Antitussive, anti-inflammatory, anti-allergy	None known
coltsfoot (*Tussilago farfara*)	Coughs, bronchitis, excessive mucus	Use for no more than two weeks at a time. Do not consume teas containing coltsfoot on a daily basis. Avoid if pregnant
damiana (*Turnera diffusa*)	Low libido, mood disorders	None known
dandelion (*Taraxacum officinale*)	Gall-bladder issues, jaundice, indigestion, muscular rheumatism, bile disturbance, poor appetite	Dandelion may increase the action of other diuretics, discuss with your health practitioner
devil's claw (*Harpagophytum procumbens*)	Arthritis, lower back pain	Avoid if you have stomach or duodenal ulcers

herb	actions/indications	contraindications
dong quai (*Angelica sinensis*)	PMS, irregular or painful periods, miscarriage, tiredness	Avoid in first three months of pregnancy
echinacea (*Echinacea purpurea*)	All types of infection, slow-healing wounds	Avoid if you have an autoimmune disease
elder (*Sambucus nigra*)	Coughs, colds and flu; anti-inflammatory	None known
elecampane (*Inula helenium*)	Upper respiratory infections, catarrh, coughs (in particular dry, irritating coughs)	None known
eyebright (*Euphrasia officinalis*)	Nasal catarrh, sinusitis, conjunctivitis (applied locally in diluted form)	Overdose can cause swelling of the eye lids
false unicorn root (*Chamaelirium luteum*)	Miscarriage, parasitic infestations, menstrual problems	Avoid if pregnant
fennel (*Foeniculum vulgare*)	Bloating, gas, colic	None known
fo-ti (*Polygonum multiflorim*)	Anti-aging, energy-boosting, cholesterol-lowering, anti-stress; good for skin conditions	None known
German chamomile (*Matricaria recutita*)	Internal: IBS, bloating, nasal catarrh, nervous diarrhea, colic, toothache, hay fever. Topical: hemorrhoids, mastitis, leg ulcers, eczema, itchy skin	Avoid if pregnant
ginger (*Zingiber officinalis*)	Lowers cholesterol, digestive aid, anti-inflammatory in arthritis (OA and RA); colic, flatulence, nausea, cold hands and feet	Avoid if taking anticoagulants
goldenseal (*Hydrastis canadensis*)	Immune-booster; food poisoning, flu, infected sinusitis, upper respiratory tract infection	Never take for more than 2 weeks at a time. Avoid with high blood pressure or if pregnant
gotu kola (*Centella asiatica*)	Memory boosting, anti-aging, healing after surgery; skin conditions, tissue regeneration	Avoid if pregnant
holy basil (*Ocimum sanctum*)	Stress, fatigue, blood-sugar maintenance	None known
horse chestnut (*Aesculus hippocastanum*)	Varicose veins, hemorrhoids, phlebitis, prostate enlargement, broken capillaries, swollen legs	Avoid if taking anticoagulants
horsetail (*Equisetum arvense*)	Wound-healing; water retention, bed wetting, cystitis	Avoid if you have kidney or heart disease
kava kava (*Piper methysticum*)	Stress, anxiety, muscular pain owing to spasms, insomnia, lower back pain	May cause headaches or vertigo. Potential to cause liver toxicity, so take daily and long term for best effects, but only for few weeks at a time before breaking (then resuming if necessary)
kigelia (*Kigelia africana*)	anti-aging, bust-firming, skin-toning and -firming; eczema, psoriasis	Use topically only (in which case no contraindications known)

herb	actions/indications	contraindications
lemon balm (*Melissa officinalis*)	Genital herpes and cold sores; insomnia, nervousness, stress, gas	None known
licorice (*Glycyrrhiza glabra*)	Bronchial catarrh, bronchitis, chronic gastritis, peptic ulcer, colic, adrenal problems (including Addison's disease), stress, estrogen imbalance	Excessive use and high doses can cause high blood pressure and water retention – avoid if suffering from either of these conditions. Check with your practitioner if on hormonal therapy
lungwort (*Pulmonaria officinalis*)	Dry hacking cough, bronchitis	None known
lycium (*Lycium barbarum*)	Immune-boosting, liver-protecting, antioxidant	None known
maca (*Lepidium meyenii*)	Increases stamina and libido in both sexes	None known
milk thistle (*Silybum marianum*)	Protects and regenerates the liver; hemorrhoids; stimulates milk flow; cancer-treatment tonic	None known
mullein (*Verbascum thapsus*)	Coughs, bronchitis, colds, flu, earache	None known
myrrh (*Commiphora myrrha*)	Colds, sinusitis, mouth ulcers, sore throats, gingivitis	Avoid if diabetic, owing to hypoglycemic action
neem (*Azadirachta indica*)	Eczema, psoriasis, dry hair, skin infections	Stick to recommended doses. Never take the oil internally (only tincture or pills)
nettle (*Urtica dioica*)	Sunburn, burns, allergies, hayfever, rashes	avoid if you have gout
nutmeg (*Myristica fragrans*)	Gas, bloating, indigestion	Use only small amounts (not more than 1 tsp a day)
oats (*Avena sativa*)	Addiction-related stress or insomnia	None known
olive leaf (*Olea europaea*)	Infections, including cold, flu, sore throat. Lowers blood pressure, helps prevent atherosclerosis	Avoid if you suffer from gall disease. If you take blood-pressure medicine, check pressure regularly
oregon grape (*Mahonia aquifolium*)	Vaginitis from bacteria or yeast; eczema, acne, psoriasis, vitiligo, herpes; gall and liver disorders	Avoid if pregnant or taking tetracyclines
passionflower (*Passiflora incarnata*)	Insomnia with exhaustion; menstrual cramps, anxiety, stress; pain relief in shingles or herpes	Avoid if taking sedatives or pregnant
pau d'arco (*Tabebuia avellanedae*)	Candida, vaginitis from bacteria or yeast, herpes, colds, flu, general infections, cancer	None known
peppermint (*Mentha piperita*)	Carminative, anti-flatulent, cooling agent, antispasmodic, analgesic, anti-fatigue	Avoid if you suffer from constipation
pine bark extract (*Pinus maritima*)	Fights damage by free radicals (antioxidant)	None known
plantain (*Plantago major*)	Cough, bronchitis, sore throat, hemorrhoids	None known
propolis (*Resina propoli*)	Wound-healing; gingivitis, sore throats, cuts, sores	None known
red clover (*Trifolium pratense*)	Eczema, psoriasis, acne, menopause	None known

herb	actions/indications	contraindications
rhodiola (*Rhodiola rosea*)	Stress, convalescence, tiredness, low immunity, improved memory and brain function	None known
rose-hip seed (*Rosa canina*)	Scars, acne scars, surgical wounds, stretch marks, post-sun pigmentation, wrinkles, radiation burns	None known
sage (*Salvia officinalis*)	Dyspepsia, pharyngitis, flatulence, gingivitis, inflammation of gums and mouth, excessive sweating; reduces milk flow	Never take sage oil internally (only the tincture). May increase action of other sedatives; avoid if pregnant, or breastfeeding (unless you want reduced milk flow)
sarsaparilla (*Smilax regelii*)	Psoriasis, rheumatism, rheumatoid arthritis	Avoid if pregnant
saw palmetto (*Serenoa rapens*)	Cystitis, prostate enlargement and other sex hormone problems	Can cause digestive symptoms such as mild diarrhea. Avoid if taking the contraceptive pill or HRT
shatavari root (*Asparagus recemosus*)	Loss of libido, infertility, miscarriage, irregular menstrual cycle	None known
skullcap (*Scutellaria lateriflora*)	Insomnia, PMS	None known
slippery elm (*Ulmus fulva*)	Coughs, stomach ulcers, gut irritation, diverticulitis, Crohn's disease	None known
St John's wort (*Hypericum perforatum*)	Anti-aging, immune-boosting; herpes (all forms), wounds (including surgical), sores, skin lesions, nerve injuries, neuralgia, depression, anxiety	May cause photosensitivity.Avoid internally if taking anticoagulants, oral contraceptives or: Cyclosporine, Digoxin, Theophyline, Indinavir
thuja (*Thuja occidentalis*)	Warts, verrucas, fungal skin infections	Not for internal use
thyme (*Thymus vulgaris*)	Antiseptic, expectorant	avoid if pregnant
triphala	Constipation, diarrhea, IBS, colitis, overweight	None known
uva ursi (*Arctostaphylos uva ursi*)	Cystitis, small kidney stones	Avoid if pregnant or breastfeeding
valerian (*Valeriana officinalis*)	Insomnia, hysterical states, migraine, cramps	Avoid if taking sedatives. Avoid alcohol, driving or operating machinery. Use for only short periods.
wild pansy (*Viola tricolor*)	Eczema, acne	None known
wild yam (*Dioscorea villosa*)	Menstrual problems and infertility, stress, menopause, kidney problems, colic	None known
willow bark (*Salix alba*)	Headaches, menstrual pain, arthritis, neuralgia, fever, colds, flu, sports injuries	Avoid if sensitive to aspirin or on aspirin therapy; or if taking anticoagulants, phenytoin or spironolactone; or if you have a gastric ulcer or are pregnant
yarrow (*Achillea millefolium*)	Wound-healing; rashes, flu	Avoid if pregnant
yellow dock (*Rumex crispus*)	Wound-healing, detoxifying; skin conditions, constipation, jaundice	Laxative – avoid excessive use; high in oxalic acid – avoid in large doses

table of supplements

supplement	actions/benefits	contraindications
alpha lipoic acid	Antioxidant both on its own and as a booster for vitamins C and E. Helps detoxify the liver, control blood sugar and protect nerve tissue	Safe and well tolerated. If diabetic, monitor your blood-sugar level closely
antioxidants	Antioxidants in general help protect our cells from oxidative damage, which contributes to heart disease, aging, degenerative diseases and cell regeneration	None known
apple cider vinegar	Antiseptic; aids digestive problems	None known
astaxanthin	A fat-soluble antioxidant that helps prevent macular degeneration, heart disease, high cholesterol, stroke, cancer and weakened immunity. A highly effective anti-inflammatory. It helps protect the skin and eyes by inhibiting damage from UVA and UVB radiation	None known
B-complex vitamins	Maintain the health of the nervous system as well as the eyes, skin, hair, mouth, muscles, gut and brain	None known
bromelain	An anti-inflammatory and digestive enzyme with anti-coagulant action	Avoid if allergic to pineapple. Not recommended for people with active gastric or duodenal ulcers. If you take anticoagulants, consult your health professional before taking bromelain supplements.
calcium	Vital for formation of bones, teeth and healthy gums. Helps keep skin and muscle healthy, lowers cholesterol and helps maintain proper cell permeability	May interfere with calcium channel blockers. Avoid if you have a history of kidney stones. Can effect absorption of certain anticonvulsants and thyroid medicines – take at least three hours apart.
chromium	Essential to help maintain blood-sugar levels. Also helps synthesize cholesterol, fats and proteins	Check with your practitioner if insulin dependent, and monitor blood-sugar levels more closely
chrondroitin	Reduces inflammation, promotes cartilage and sustains elasticity in skin, joints and blood-vessel walls	None known
co-enzyme Q10	An antioxidant that helps to produce energy within cells but also helps boost immunity, circulation and gum health. An excellent anti-aging vitamin	None known
cranberry	Helps prevent and treat urinary tract infections. Rich in antioxidants	None known
detox capsules	A mixture of green foods, herbs and clay designed to cleanse the gut. Also helps reduce toxicity	None known. Drink 6–8 glasses of water daily if taking detox capsules
digestive enzymes	A mixture of amylase, protease and lipase to aid digestion of carbohydrates, proteins and fats	If you have an active stomach ulcer, take these only with meals and with advice from a health professional
essential fatty acids (EFAs)	Help maintain healthy skin, hair and nerves. Cholesterol-lowering, anti-inflammatory and hormone-balancing	None known

supplement	actions/benefits	contraindications
glucosamine	Helps treat osteoarthritis and maintain skin health	None known
grapefruit seed extract	Antimicrobial agent excellent for treating candidiasis and general food poisoning	None known. If also taking cholesterol-lowering medication or anti-histamines take at least 2 hours apart
hydrochloric acid (betain hydrochloride)	Helps digestion and to prevent the proliferation of pathogens that enter the body through food or drink	Consult your practitioner if suffering from a gastric or duodenal ulcer or if taking a non-steroidal anti-inflammatory drug
L lysine	Useful against herpes (genital and cold sores)	None known
linseed	May help prevent blood clots, high blood pressure, PMS, skin and other inflammation (arthritis, eczema). Necessary for brain growth. Helps keep bowels healthy	None known. Grind seeds before using them otherwise they will go straight through the system. Take seeds away from any medication or supplements
magnesium	Helps with insomnia, muscle cramps, PMS, bone formation, constipation and high blood pressure	Avoid if taking Amiloride, Ciprofloxacin, Sulfonyureas, Tetracycline or Warfarin; or if you have kidney failure
MSM	Helps nourish hair, skin and nails; detoxifying	None known
oligomeric proanthocyanidins	Powerful antioxidants that protect cells, skin, brain and nerves from free radicals; liver protecting	None known
potassium	Helps nerve and muscle health, and to maintain correct water balance in the body	If you have a kidney disorder, take potassium only under the advice of your healthcare professional
probiotics	Inhibit bad bacteria; promote digestion and immunity; help lactose sensitivity, IBS, skin problems and candida	None known
quercetin	Anti-inflammatory so helps in allergic conditions	None known
red marine algae	Antiviral, particularly against herpes	None known
selenium	Mineral antioxidant. Also helps protect immune system and is needed for fat metabolism and thyroid function. Known to protect the liver from alcohol cirrhosis	None known
vitamin A	Antioxidant. Good for eyes, lungs and skin, new cell growth and in the treatment of wrinkles	Best taken as betacarotene. If you are pregnant, avoid in high doses (over 10,000iu)
vitamin (ester) C	A multi-purpose antioxidant for tissue repair, immune function, detoxification, lowering cholesterol and collagen formation. Ester C is the non-acidic version	Large doses of acidic vitamin C (that is, not ester C) can cause stomach irritation
vitamin E	Antioxidant. Helps protect skin, nerves and muscles and prevent PMS, high blood pressure and heart disease	None known
zinc	Helps heal the skin and regulates sebum production. Protects the health of the prostate gland in men	Never take zinc at the same time as an iron supplement, as they affect each other's absorption

visual index of plants

All the images in this glossary appear elsewhere in this book. The plants are organized according to the order in which these images first appear. **Bold** numbers refer to plants with full-page plant portrait images.

Bilberry
(*Vaccinium myrtillus*)
pp.19, 197

Eucalyptus
pp.19, 78

Licorice
(*Glycyrrhiza glabra*) pp.19, 46, 79, **103**, 105

Rhodiola
(*Rhodiola rosea*)
pp.19, 113

Psyllium
(*Plantago psyllium*) p.46

Linseed
(*Linum usitatissimum, Linaceae*) pp.46, **83**

Alfalfa
(*Medicago sativa*)
p.46

Milk thistle
(*Sylibum marianum*)
pp.49, 87

Dandelion
(*Taraxacum officinale*)
pp.49, 159

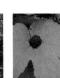

Red clover
(*Trifolium pratense*)
pp.49, 135, 164

Artichoke
(*Cynara scolymus*)
pp.**24**, 49

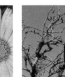

Plantain
(*Plantago major*)
pp.60, 75

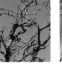

St John's wort
(*Hypericum perforatum*)
pp.60, 71, 123, **125**, 136, 138, 149, 175

Olive leaf
(*Olea europaea*)
pp.60, 87, **89**, 95, 136, **168**, 175

Lemon balm
(*Melissa officinalis*)
pp.60, 136, 137

Thyme
(*Thymus vulgaris*)
p.63

Yarrow
(*Achillea millefolium*)
p.65

Peppermint
(*Mentha piperita*)
pp.**56**, 65, 80, 91, 105

Astragalus
(*Astragalus membranaceus*)
pp.65, 75, 163

Goldenseal
(*Hydrastis canadensis*)
pp.65, 87, 95, 136

Sage
(*Salvia officinalis*)
pp.67, **167**

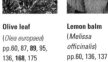

Calendula
(*Calendula officinalis*)
pp.67, 123, 126, 135, 149, 175, 197

Myrrh
(*Commiphora myrrha*)
p.67

Echinacea
(*Echinacea purpurea*)
pp.**59**, 67, 75, 95

Mullein
(*Verbascum thapsus*)
p.75

Elecampane
(*Inula helenium*)
p.79

Coltsfoot
(*Tussilago farfara*)
p.79

Lungwort
(*Pulmonaria officinalis*)
pp.**77**, 79

Anise
(*Pimpinella anisum*)
p.80

Fennel
(*Foeniculum vulgare*)
pp.80, **171**

Ginger
(*Zingiber officinalis*)
pp.80, 87, 91, **116**, 119

German chamomile
(*Matricaria recutita*)
pp.91, 99, 111, 141

Aloe vera
(*Aloe vera*)
pp.91, 105, 106, 123, 135, 175

Pau d'arco
(*Tabebuia avellanedae*)
p.95

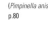

Eyebright
(*Euphrasia officinalis*)
p.98

Elderflower
(*Sambucus nigra*)
pp.**92**, 99

Nettle
(*Urtica dioica*)
p.99

Grasses
pp.99, **101**

Slippery elm
- (*Ulmus fulva*)
p.105

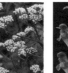

Oats
(*Avena sativa*)
pp.111, 163

Valerian
(*Valeriana officinalis*)
pp.**109**, 111

Skullcap
(*Scutellaria lateriflora*)
pp.111, 159

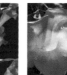

Devil's claw
(*Harpagophytum procumbens*) p.119

Black cohosh
(*Cimicifuga racemosa*)
pp.119, 164

Willow bark
(*Salix alba*)
p.119

Gotu kola
(*Centella asiatica*)
pp.123, 149, 197

Horse chestnut
(*Aesculus hippocastanum*)
p.129

Burdock
(*Arctium lappa*)
p.**133**

Rose geranium
(*Pelargonium* 'Graveolens') p.134

Tea tree
(*Melaleuca alternifolia*)
pp.135, 177

Chickweed
(*Stellaria media*)
p.141

Neem
(*Azadirachta indica*)
pp.141, 145

Wild Pansy
(*Viola tricolor*)
pp.141, 145

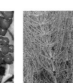

Lycium
(*Lycium barbarum*)
p.145

Sarsaparilla
(*Smilax regelii*)
p.145

Horsetail
(*Equisetum arvense*)
p.149

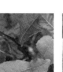

Rose hip
(*Rosa canina*)
pp.150, 174

Agnus castus
(*Vitex agnus castus*)
pp.157, 159, 160

Evening primrose
(*Oenothera biennis*)
pp.**143**, 159

False unicorn root (*Chamaelirium luteum*)
p.160

Shatavari root
(*Asparagus racemosus*)
p.160

Wild yam
(*Dioscorea villosa*)
p.160

Flannel flower
(*Actinotus helianthi*)
p.162

Saw palmetto
(*Serenoa repens*)
p.163

Fo-ti
(*Polygonium multiflorim*)
p.163

Dong quai
(*Angelica sinensis*)
p.164

Damiana
(*Turnera diffusa*)
p.164

Kigelia
(*Kigelia africana*)
p.197

Green tea
(*Camellia sinensis*)
p.198

Rose
(*Rosa damascena*)
pp.**180**, 200

visual index of foods

All the images in this glossary appear elsewhere in this book. The foods are organized according to the order in which these images first appear. **Bold** numbers refer to foods with full-page portrait images.

Asparagus
p.15

Curly endive
p.15

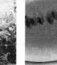
Watermelon
p.15

Cranberry
p.15

Alfalfa
pp.20, **130**

Kiwi
p.20

Sesame seeds
p.20

Yogurt
pp.20, 97

Artichoke
pp.**24**, 34

Tumeric
p.34

Rosemary
p.34

Celery
pp.34

Pineapple
pp.35, 121

Beetroot
p.35

Watercress
pp.35, 155

Pear
p.35

Lentils
p.85

Nuts
p.85

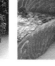
Apple
p.85

Kale
p.85

Salmon
pp.97, 115, 191

Oats
pp.97

Quinoa
p.97

Tofu
p.115

Brown rice
p.115

Berries
p.115

Garlic
p.155

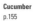
Parsley
p.155

Cucumber
p.155

Orange
p.191

Green tea
p.191

Broccoli
p.191

Wheatgrass
p.**193**

Lemon
p.195

index

acknowledgments

The publisher would like to thank the following photographic libraries and Deni Bown for permission to reproduce their material. Any errors or omissions are entirely unintentional and the publishers will, if informed, make amendments in future editions of this book:

Abbreviations:
DB = Deni Bown, DBP = Duncan Baird Publishers' archive

Inside cover & page **1**: Valentina Petrova/Getty Images; **15** DBP; **19** DB, Peter Anderson/ Dorling Kindersley/Getty Images, DB, DB; **20** DBP; **30** David Noble/Getty Images; **32** PM Images/Getty Images; **33** Andy Sacks/Getty Images; **34** DBP; **35** DBP; **37** DBP; **46** DB; **49** DB, Matt Anker/Getty Images, DB, Comet/Corbis; **59** DBP; **60** Deni Bown/Dorling Kindersley, DB, DB, DB; **63** DB; **65** DB; **67** DB; **71** DB; **72–73** Alamy Images; **75** DB/Dorling Kindersley, Mark Bolton/Corbis, DB, DB; **78** Peter Anderson/Dorling Kindersley/Getty Images; **79** DB; **80** Science Photo Library, DB, DB, DB; **85** DBP; **87** DB; **91** DB, DB, DB, DBP; **95** DB; **97** DBP; **98** DB; **99** DB, DB, DB, Herbert Zetti/Corbis; **101** Herbert Zetti/Corbis; **105** DBP, DB, DB, DB; **106–7** DBP; **111** DB, DB, TH Foto/Photolibrary, DB; **113** DB; **115** DBP; **119** DB; **121** DBP; **123** DB, DB, DBP; **126–7** DB; **129** Ian Beames/Corbis; **134** Roger Smith/Dorling Kindersley; **135** DB, DB, DBP, DB; **136** DB; **137** DB; **138–139** DB; **141** DB; **145** DB, DB, DB, Bruno Petriglia/Science Photo Library; **149** DB; **150–151** DB; **155** DBP;

157 Bruno Petriglia/Science Photo Library; **159** DB, TH FOTO/Photolibrary, Mark Anker/Getty Images, DB; **160** Steve Gorton/Dorling Kindersley, DB, DB, DB; **162** Ken Griffiths/NHPA; **163** W. Perry Conway/Corbis, DB, Lew Robertson/Getty Images, DB; **164** DB, DB, DB, Andy Crawford & Steve Gorton/Dorling Kindersley; **173** DBP; **174** Deni Bown; **175** DB, DBP, DB, DB; **177** DB; **191** DBP; **193** DBP; **195** DBP; **197** DB; **198** DB; **200–201** DEA RANDOM/Getty Images; **210** DBP

Commissioned Photography:
Toby Scott: **4–5, 6–7, 17, 24, 51, 53, 54–55, 56, 69, 77, 83, 89, 92, 103, 109, 116, 125, 130, 133, 143, 152, 167, 168, 171, 180, 188**
Jules Selmes: **13, 39, 41, 44, 185, 189**

Publisher's acknowledgments: The publisher would like to thank Arne Herbs and Jekka's Herbs for supplying plants for the photoshoot, and The Organic Herb Trading Company for advice and supplying fresh rose petals. They would also like to thank model Sarina Carruthers and make-up artist Justine Martin, and food stylist Jennie Shapter.

Author's acknowledgments: I'd like to thank Grace Cheetham and Roger Walton for making this happen; my husband who is my rock; and my children Roksana and Maxi who keep me young.